Howell Equine Handbook

of **Tendon** and **Ligament Injuries**

Linda B. Schultz, DVM, PhD

HOWELL
BOOK
HOUSE

Howell Equine Handbook

Howell Equine Handbook

of **Tendon** and **Ligament Injuries**

Linda B. Schultz, DVM, PhD

HOWELL
BOOK
HOUSE

For Ryan, the greatest of God's gifts, for mommy's part of the castle.

Howell Book House
Published by Wiley Publishing, Inc., Hoboken, New Jersey

Published simultaneously in Canada

For general information on our other products and services or to obtain technical support please contact our Customer Care Department within the U.S. at (800) 762-2974, outside the United States at (317) 572-3993 or fax (317) 572-4002.

Wiley also publishes its books in a variety of electronic formats. Some content that appears in print may not be available in electronic books. For more information about Wiley products, visit our web site at www.wiley.com.

Library of Congress Cataloging-in-Publication Data:
Schultz, Linda B., date.
  Howell equine handbook : tendon and ligament injuries in the horse / Linda B. Schultz.
     p. cm.
Includes bibliographical references and index.
  ISBN 0-7645-7435-3 (cloth : alk. paper)—ISBN 0-7645-5715-7 (pbk. : alk. paper)
1. Tendons—Wounds and injuries. 2. Ligaments—Wounds and injuries.
3. Horses—Wounds and injuries. I. Title: Tendon and ligament injuries in the horse. II. Title.
  SF959.T47S36 2004
  636.1'0897474044—dc22

Printed in the United States of America

10   9   8   7   6   5   4   3   2   1

Contents

Acknowledgments

Books are the culmination of many people's efforts, each effort placed differently in the life of the writer and each required for a successful product. My life is blessed with many gifted individuals without whom this book, and my entire writing career, would not be. I thank my husband, Kevin Schultz, my biggest supporter and consummate encourager, for compelling me to follow my heart. I thank Susan Aiello for nuturing my writing efforts. To my agent, Jacky Sach, thank you for "finding" me and waiting for the mystery. I thank my editors Dale Cunningham and Maggie Bonham for guidance through the publishing maze, and Sharon Sakson for giving her all at the end. Two expert veterinary consultants, Steve Trostle, DVM, MS, and Mary Beth Whitcomb, DVM, graciously provided beautiful photographs and technical information where progress in equine practice had outpaced my reading. Allison Howell, DVM, and Ed Boldt, DVM, kindly provided firsthand information about acupuncture and chiropractic care in horses amidst their busy equine practices. I thank Allison Wright, MS, CMI, for her prompt and competent illustrative services. My family could not have survived this book without the dedication of Jackie Costa and her family even in the midst of Israel's premature yet enchanting entrance into this world. Thank you for loving us so much and helping me see my path. Love and special thanks go to my best writing friends and mentors Jean Adair, Steve Brown, Jeffrey Phillips and Jim Frey for understanding what only other writers understand and for always being there. God has placed each of these precious people in my life for which I thank Him. With God, through Jesus Christ, all things are possible.

Introduction

Injuries to the lower legs' tendons and ligaments are the most common medical conditions horses suffer. You know this if you raise, train or care for an equine athlete. The severity ranges from minor injuries to those that end careers or even the horse's life. You try to prevent these injuries every day with wraps, support boots and different workout schedules. Yet despite all the research and experience of the equine veterinary and lay community, no one really knows how to do this.

But there is hope. We've seen changes in treatment, new medications, diagnostic ultrasound and other inventions that have revolutionized diagnosis and care. These modern treatments, along with controlled exercise, help horses heal safely and return to work more often than in the past. A horse with tendon and ligament injuries can make a full recovery, depending on the injury and care.

This guidebook will help you learn more about tendon and ligament injuries. The book discusses anatomy, how and why tendon and ligament injuries occur and the principles of common therapies. You'll see a sample controlled exercise schedule and guidelines for recuperation times. You'll understand your horse's condition and why the care works. You'll learn the importance of talking with your veterinarian so your horse will be back on his feet and hopefully doing his job, whether it's racing, jumping, dressage, roping, team penning or another equine sport. Your relationship with your veterinarian is very important for your horse's recuperation.

Go in knowledge.

Chapter 1

Diagnosing Tendon and Ligament Injuries

If you're reading this book, you either have a lame horse who's been diagnosed with a tendon or ligament injury, or a knowledgeable stablemate, trainer or other "horse person" has told you that your horse has a tendon or ligament problem. Regardless of your level of expertise, this book will help you fill in the gaps, understand your horse's condition and help you through the phases of healing. Whether you have pleasure horses, racehorses, hunters, jumpers, dressage horses or trail horses, you will understand more about their legs and how they work once you've consulted this book. You need to be as informed as possible about your animal's health care, especially in conditions that can be as severe and career-ending as tendon and ligament disorders.

Most common tendon and ligament injuries can be quite serious. Many racehorses who injure a tendon or ligament will not race again. Other athletes may not return to their previous level of performance. However, the same horse may make a nice hunter or trail horse. Most injuries occur in the foreleg because the horse bears almost 70 percent of his weight there. The most common injury occurs to the superficial digital flexor tendon (SDF; one of the major tendons on the back of the foreleg—more on this in Chapter 2,

"Functional Anatomy of the Equine Foreleg and Hind Leg"), followed by injury to the deep digital flexor tendon (DDF) and suspensory ligament. Each has similar findings at the cellular level and requires almost identical treatment regimes. When you understand what happens inside the tendon you'll understand why your veterinarian has prescribed certain therapies. Working with your vet is very important to a successful recovery from this or any injury.

Working with Your Veterinarian

Good communication with your vet is important when treating your horse, even if you have a trainer working with the veterinarian. Your information may be secondhand and may be garbled. Ask your vet any questions you might have and clarify the diagnosis and treatment.

Your vet should be happy to answer your questions. In fact, most vets prefer to talk more about the condition because your interest shows you are a conscientious owner. If your vet doesn't want to discuss your horse's condition, you should ask why and perhaps look for another vet. A good vet is patient and willing to discuss information on the level you're comfortable with.

Tendon Injury at the Cellular Level

Tendon injuries come in all sizes and degrees. They may be subclinical—so small that they cannot be detected without ultrasound—or they may be a complete tendon rupture. Inflammation, a complex process involving the immune system, occurs after an injury and is the first step to healing. Blood vessel dilation and leakiness, swelling, heat, pain and an increase of inflammatory blood cells are all signs of beginning inflammation. The goal of therapy, as we'll see soon, is to aggressively decrease inflammation. We'll discuss more about this later in this chapter and in Chapter 4.

A horse that limps from the track or arena with a tendon injury usually has swelling, hemorrhage (bleeding) into the lesion and tendon edema (internal swelling of the tendon) from inflammation. Fluid leaks into the tendon and, along with the blood, separates and weakens the remaining normal fibers. The body tries to clean up the damaged tissue by releasing enzymes, called *hydrolytic enzymes,* that would normally chew up damaged tissue into smaller sizes that can be carried away by the circulation. In excess, they can cause further damage to the collagen fibers and the glue that holds the fibers together, the interfibrillar matrix. In the process of the injury, the horse may have damaged the blood vessels, which may lead to *necrosis* (cell death).

Recognizing Tendon or Ligament Injury

Although you should have your veterinarian diagnose any suspected tendon or ligament injuries, these injuries are not difficult to spot. There are characteristic clues that with some help and practice you will be able observe.

Visually Examining Your Horse

You don't have to be a vet to detect injuries. Most animals with even a moderate tendon or ligament injury will be obviously lame. It's the more subtle injuries, the ones that might happen before the "big" one that you can train yourself to look for in your horse. A daily examination should be a routine every time you train or ride your horse.

Look at your horse's legs every day while he's uninjured both before and after you ride or train. By learning what normal looks like, you might be able to detect what looks abnormal. If your horse wears boots, use the moment before applying them to scan his lower limb for any sign of swelling, heat or thickening. Being familiar with your horse's legs will help you identify problems before they have a chance to worsen.

SIGNS OF TENDON OR LIGAMENT INJURY

- Lameness
- Heat
- Swelling
- Pain on touch

You won't be able to detect all injuries, but you'll have a good chance at recognizing severe, moderate and maybe even mild tendon and ligament injuries when you examine your horse every day.

Lameness

Horses with mild injuries may not be noticeably limping, or lame. But most horses with at least moderate tendon or ligament injuries will be lame. In the case of a severe injury, you'll see that the horse is not bearing weight on a leg or is severely bobbing his head while walking.

Even though not all horses with tendon or ligament injuries are lame, there may be other signs present that the owner may or may not recognize. Talk with your vet if you suspect something is wrong with your horse's gait. Your vet can examine your horse for lameness. Diagnosing the cause of lameness, especially mild lameness, requires the experience and training of a veterinarian.

A horse who is intermittently lame can be frustrating. One day you ride and he is "off"; the next he's fine. Another day, you ride in deep sand and he's lame. The next day he seems off going one direction but not the other. What's important is that he is lame and your vet should examine him. There is no other answer for this problem. Mild tendon or ligament injuries that cause intermittent lameness will eventually become a big problem. The time, effort and money spent to correctly diagnose the problem are well worth it.

Swelling

Swelling is a common sign of acute tendon and ligament injuries. Inflammation causes blood vessels to dilate (enlarge). The blood vessel leaks fluid into the surrounding tissue and causes swelling. Hemorrhage (bleeding) into the tissue can also cause swelling. Swelling of the SDF tendon causes the "bowed" appearance of a horse's lower leg in a "bowed" tendon (see Figure 1).

Although swelling is a common sign of tendon or ligament injury, not all injuries will result in swelling or it may be slight. Being familiar with what looks normal for your horse's legs is important in detecting slight swelling.

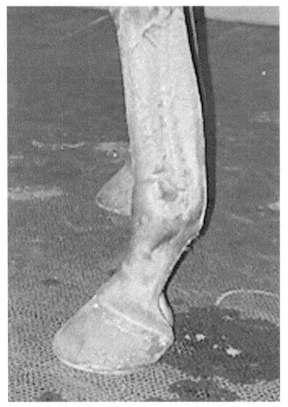

Fig. 1. A bowed tendon.

Pain on Touch (Palpation)

Tendon and ligament injuries hurt. The inflammatory process following an injury causes heat and pain. You can detect the pain through *palpation* (feeling your horse's injured leg with your fingers). Veterinarians and horse owners can gently palpate a horse's tendons and ligaments to determine his pain level. This takes practice and knowledge of anatomy, which is covered in the next chapter.

Many horses don't like their tendons or ligaments palpated (especially their suspensory ligament) while standing. Palpating an injured leg while the horse is standing on it can be inconclusive. You may have anything from no reaction to rearing up, depending on the horse and the injury. But an injured horse will usually react to palpation if the leg isn't bearing weight.

HOW TO PALPATE YOUR HORSE'S TENDONS

Hold your horse's hoof in one hand while palpating the tendons with the other. Start at the top, just below the knee, and gently work your fingers inch by inch down one tendon, say the SDF tendon. Then do the same for the DDF tendon and then the suspensory ligament. It is not only a good way to feel for pain, but also deep swelling, thickening and heat. If your horse reacts to palpation, it doesn't necessarily mean he has pain.

Although palpation is valuable, it requires palpating hundreds of injured and noninjured horses to really get a feel for this. One key is to palpate the opposite leg for a comparison. Comparing the legs can give you a much better reading on your horse's pain level. If you get the same reaction on the other side, either you have two problems (unlikely) or none at all. Another key is knowing your horse's anatomy (see Chapter 2).

Heat

Inflammation often causes heat because of blood vessel dilation. The inflammation causes more blood to circulate through the region and causes the area to be warmer. Studies show that only about 20 percent of horses with tendon or ligament injury have increased heat in the affected leg. Therefore, heat is used moderately to assess tendon and ligament injuries.

But heat isn't something that you should ignore. If you feel heat in your horse's tendons, have your vet evaluate him for injury.

Diagnosis

Diagnosing a tendon or ligament injury requires a trained veterinarian. However, you can assist your vet with the proper diagnosis. One way is to provide the vet with a detailed and accurate history. Your vet will want to know your horse's age and training competition level. Your vet will also need to know when your horse was injured, what activity precluded the injury, the horse's conditioning schedule, all medications (if any) administered to the horse prior to his examination and all therapies administered such as cold water hosing, bandaging, poultices applied or ice baths. He or she will also want to know if the horse was on stall rest or in a paddock. Your vet will then begin the lameness exam.

Lameness Exam

Depending on your horse's injury, the lameness exam can be very short or quite extensive. A horse who has an obvious injury such as a bowed tendon will require less exam time than a horse with a mild high suspensory ligament injury, which requires more time to diagnose. The veterinarian notes the horse's conformation, noting hoof wear and shoeing; observing all joints, tendons and ligaments of the lower leg; and visually inspecting back, rump and leg muscles for swelling or atrophy (degeneration). The vet should examine each hoof and should apply hoof testers to rule out any foot abnormalities.

Your vet should rule out each abnormality found during this initial exam as a cause of lameness during the exercise and palpation part of the exam.

After the initial exam, your veterinarian will ask you or an assistant to walk and trot your horse in a straight line and in circles in both directions. The handler's role is critical here. Hold the horse loosely so that his head is centered in line with his body. If you hold his head too tightly, your vet may not catch any subtle head nodding. If your horse is lame in one of the forelegs, your horse will drop his head (nod or bob) when he steps with the sound foot and raise his head when he steps with the unsound foot. This can be tricky, but if you think about when you stub a toe or step barefoot on a stone, you tend to lift your body when your sore foot hits the ground to get as much weight as possible off that foot. A horse will do the same thing. Therefore, his head will move up in an exaggerated manner when his sore foot hits the ground. If your vet can't detect lameness while the horse walks, then you must trot your horse. Your vet can detect lameness more easily when the horse is trotting because at any one time the horse only has two feet on the ground, which will distribute more of his body weight to the injured leg, making the lameness more apparent.

HOOF TESTERS

A hoof tester is a large instrument that looks like an unusual set of pliers. Veterinarians use hoof testers to apply pressure in a systematic manner to the entire sole and frog region of the hoof to identify any region of sensitivity that might be cause for lameness.

Determining subtle lameness in the hind legs is more complicated. Your vet will tell you how to move your horse so he can
detect the lameness.

A horse with a bowed tendon will be noticeably lame at a walk
and the "bow" will be obvious. A horse with a less severe injury
might only be lame at a trot on concrete in circles to the right.
Depending on the severity of the injury, it may require more time
to diagnose.

Lameness is graded on a scale of Grade 1 (least lame) to Grade
4 (most lame). The vet grades the lameness so that he or she has a
reference point at each visit. This grading is useful to other vets if
they treat your horse. This grading is also important to determine
if there's improvement or worsening.

Once your vet identifies the unsound leg, he or she will palpate
the lower leg to isolate the problem. Your vet should palpate all
joints, tendons and ligaments and note abnormalities. The problem
may be obvious or perplexing. In less obvious injuries, the vet may
wish to conduct other tests.

Diagnostic Tests

Most times, your veterinarian will need to perform one or more
diagnostic tests to accurately diagnose your horse's lameness.
Some tests are part of the lameness examination and some are in
addition to the exam and will be an additional expense. However, it
is worth knowing exactly what is wrong with your horse so that you
can get on the road to recovery.

Flexion Tests

Flexion tests assist your vet in identifying joint problems and may
be useful in diagnosing tendon or ligament injuries as well. In a
flexion test of the fetlock joint, the vet bends and holds the joint
with moderate pressure for at least one minute. Then you trot the

horse. If the horse is lame in the fetlock joint, he will be noticeably lamer following this test. However, the flexor tendons are also crimped together, which may worsen the lameness along with any fetlock joint problems. This is especially true for horses with injured DDF tendons (see Figure 2).

A positive flexion test may still mean the tendons or ligaments are involved. Your veterinarian may rule out fetlock joint problems by using a local anesthetic to block nerves in the lower leg, called a *local anesthetic nerve block.*

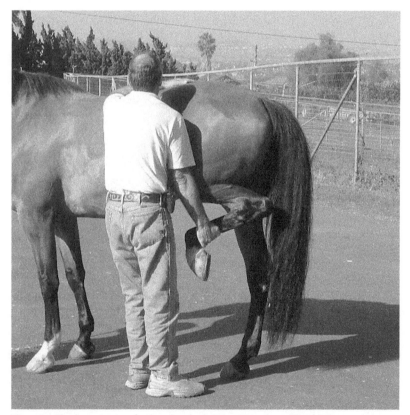

Fig. 2. Flexion test of the hock joint. Horses with high suspensory ligament desmitis, such as occurs often in Standardbred racehorses, will have positive hock flexion tests in 85 percent of hind-limb cases.

LOCAL ANESTHETIC NERVE BLOCKS

Vets use nerve blocks to eliminate feeling in a region of the horse's leg so that they can locate the lameness. For example, if you have a horse with swollen tendons who is positive to hoof testers in the same leg, you may not be able to determine whether his pain is coming from his foot or his tendons. In this case, the nerves that serve the foot can be isolated and blocked with a local anesthetic. If the horse trots off sound, you know the lameness is coming from his foot and not his swollen tendons. The tendons may need care as well, but this test can isolate the cause of lameness. If he trots off noticeably improved but is still lame, you know that part of his lameness may be coming from his tendons.

Diagnosis is a little more complicated than that, but this is what your veterinarian is doing when he "blocks" your horse.

Thermography

Thermography is used to measure and record temperatures in a horse's leg. Vets and researchers thought it was useful in subclinical cases where the animal showed no lameness. Although it was popular in the mid- to late 1990s, it is seldom used today.

Thermography is very sensitive to changes in surface temperatures, but not very specific. For example, a leg under a bandage may appear "hot" on a thermographic study. A horse standing in a barn aisle with one side to an open door could have different thermographic studies between the two sides. There is a lot of potential for artifact interpretation with thermography and it most likely only measures what is going on at the surface and not what's happening in deeper tissues. Therefore, thermography has limited value in diagnosing a tendon or ligament injury.

Ultrasound

Diagnostic ultrasound has truly revolutionized the diagnosing and monitoring of tendon and ligament injuries in the horse. In fact, a vet can't fully or accurately diagnose a tendon or ligament injury without an ultrasound exam (see Figure 3).

An ultrasound image is formed when ultrasound waves (sound waves) applied to the tendon reflect back from the tissues. The

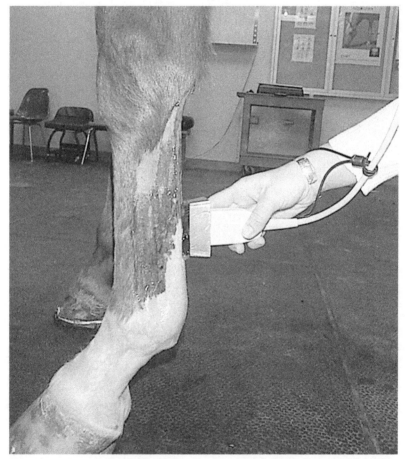

Fig. 3. An ultrasound examination of the tendons of the forelimb. This picture shows the ultrasound probe.

reflected waves are converted to an electrical impulse that is displayed on a small screen. The image is caused by differences in the tissues' ability to reflect the wave. Because there aren't many structures in the horse's leg, it's easy for a trained eye to read the ultrasound.

Tissues of different densities will cause the image to appear either darker (almost black) or lighter (white). For example, bone, the most dense, appears white on ultrasound. The tendons appear gray and fluid such as blood or water appears black. A lesion in a tendon will appear darker than the surrounding tendon because the injury makes the region less dense and there is fluid or blood (see Figure 4).

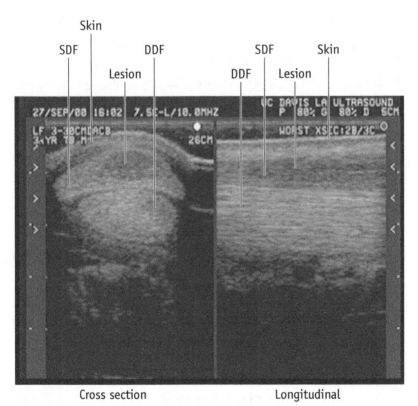

Fig. 4. A moderate tear of the SDF tendon in a cross section and longitudinally.

Note that an ultrasonigraphic assessment performed on the first day after the injury may not show the full severity of the injury. Ideally, performing an ultrasound examination four or five days after the injury will show the full extent of the damage. Ultrasound is also invaluable for monitoring the progress of healing before moving the horse to the next level of work. We'll discuss using ultrasound for rehabilitation in Chapter 4.

Radiographs (X-rays)

Radiographs (X-rays) are most useful for diagnosing bony conditions that could lead to lameness. Tissues such as tendons and ligaments do not readily appear on radiographs, making their use in diagnosing tendon and ligament injuries minimal. However, they're helpful in avulsion fractures in which a tendon or ligament has pulled away from the bone and pulled some of the bone with it. The vet can see the bone chips on an X-ray. Avulsion fractures can occur at the suspensory ligament's point of origin in the back and base of the horse's knee or at the paired sesamoid bones where the branch of the suspensory ligament lies. Fractures of the paired splint bones that heal inadequately can also cause problems with the suspensory ligament.

In Summary

- Make sure you are comfortable with your veterinarian and feel at ease to ask questions.

- Tendon and ligament injury results in inflammation, which includes blood vessel dilation and leaking, swelling, heat and pain.

- Not all horses who have a tendon or ligament injury are lame.

- Diagnostic ultrasound is the gold standard of diagnostic tests.

- Proper diagnosis requires your veterinarian so that the nature and extent of the injuries are fully evaluated.

Chapter 2

Functional Anatomy of the Equine Foreleg and Hind Leg

Knowing your horse's anatomy is the first step to understanding tendon and ligament injuries. It's important to know the structure's location and function to appreciate how it works, why it breaks down and how it heals. Although horses have tendons and ligaments throughout their bodies, those of the lower leg are the most prone to injury.

Tendons

Tendons make it possible for your horse to stand up, sleep, walk, run, jump and play. This section covers how tendons work and what they're made of, and will give you some specifics on anatomy. Anatomy will help you understand your horse's injury and allow you to work with your veterinarian more closely.

FUNCTION OF TENDONS

Tendons have three primary functions:

- Flexion or extension of joints
- Support and stabilization of joints
- Shock absorption

Function

Tendons connect muscle to bone. They are commonly confused with *ligaments*, which connect bone with bone. (We'll discuss ligaments in the next section.) Tendons have three major functions in the body:

1. Skeletal movement, either *flexion* or *extension.* Muscles are attached to the skeleton by tendons and contract to produce skeletal movement. An example of flexion is when the back muscles of your horse's foreleg contract, he can flex his *fetlock joint* (the equivalent of bending your wrist down and attempting to touch your fingers to the forearm's underside) because tendons attach the muscle to the lower leg bones. Extension is the opposite of flexion. It is the equivalent of bending your wrist up toward your forearm and uses the opposing muscles and tendons.

2. Support and stabilization. Tendons provide support to joints (where bone meets bone), which stabilizes them, or makes them unable to come apart easily. Your entire horse's weight bears down on seven bones and three major joints below the knee. You can see that stabilization is vital in this area, even when the horse is at rest. But in the equine athlete, joint stabilization is critical when he's expected to jump oxers, race around barrels, scramble after a calf or perform intricate footwork.

3. Shock absorption and recoiling. Tendons also provide a type of shock absorption, like a car's suspension. Look at the close-up photo of a racehorse's fetlock while weight-bearing at a full run (see Figure 5). In this, you can see the flexibility and shock-absorbing qualities of tendons at work. Although overextension of the fetlock joint depicted in this photo can result in chip fractures, it shows the tendons' flexibility. The tendons recoil and assist the horse, pulling his leg up and forward for the next step.

Tendons are dense bands of fibrous connective tissue (a common tissue throughout the body). Fascicles, tiny bundles of Type I collagen fibrils (the protein that provides tendon strength) make up the tendon. Other proteins, elastic fibers, water and fibroblasts (cells that make collagen) fill the spaces between fascicles. *Peritendon,* a thin layer of tissue, surrounds each fascicle, holding the individual collagen fibers together. *Epitendon,* another thin layer of tissue, surrounds groups of fascicles to form the tendon unit (see Figure 6). The tendon structure looks like a rope. Smaller fibers are bundled into larger bundles, which then are bundled to

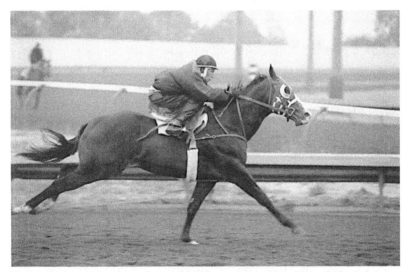

Fig. 5. Thoroughbred racehorse with hyperextension of the fetlock joint.

DEFINITIONS

Flexion: the act of bending a joint using the flexor muscles. For example, bending your wrist down, or your horse's knee and fetlock when you pick up his foot to clean his hoof.

Extension: the act of bending a joint using the extensor muscles. For example, bending your wrist up, or when your horse's leg is extended forward.

Fetlock: the first joint below your horse's knee and hock joints.

Stabilization: the act of making a joint stable. For example, a stack of blocks glued together are more stable than those simply resting on one another.

---

form the final rope. Besides holding the bundles and the fascicles together, the epitendon and peritendon are connective tissues that carry blood vessels, supplying blood to the inside of the tendon.

A tendon may have a tendon sheath where the tendon slides over joints, such as the fetlock joint. The tendon sheath supplies blood to the external tendon. The tendon sheath also secretes *synovial* fluid, a thick, slippery substance that aids the tendon in gliding over joints. A thin connective tissue called *paratendon* (notice that this is different from peritendon) surrounds unsheathed tendons. The paratendon also facilitates tendon gliding and supplies blood to the external part of the tendon.

There are four potential sources of blood supply to the tendon: the muscle, the bone, the synovial sheath (if present) and the paratendon (if no sheath exists). Muscle and bone supply the distal (outer) 25 percent of the tendon, with the remaining 75 percent of the tendon being supplied by vessels from the sheath or paratendon. It is important to understand the tendon's blood supply because tendon healing requires blood to supply oxygen and nutrients. Without the blood supply, the tissue will die.

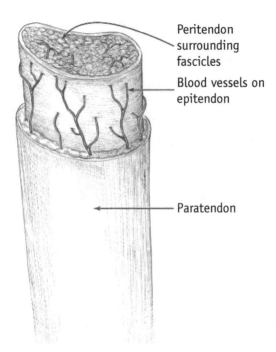

Peritendon surrounding fascicles

Blood vessels on epitendon

Paratendon

Fig. 6. A cross section of an equine tendon.

Ligaments

Ligaments connect bone to bone. The suspensory ligament is the most commonly injured ligament in the horse. As in the tendon section, here we discuss the function and composition of ligaments.

Function

Ligaments are bands of fibrous tissue that connect bones or cartilages. They support the musculoskeletal system. Unlike tendons, they do not assist in movement, but instead they stabilize a horse's joints. Imagine stacking children's blocks the way a horse's lower leg bones are stacked and then trying to sit on the top block. The stack would buckle. However, if you ran strong bands between the blocks and connected them at the joints, you might have a tower strong enough to hold your weight. This is how ligaments hold joints together to support your horse's weight. Some ligaments, such as the *suspensory* ligament along the back of the cannon bone (the large bone below the horse's knee), also function to absorb shock, like tendons.

The ligaments' names usually refer to their location on the joint. Ligaments that are on the joint's sides (the lateral aspect) are called *collateral ligaments*. Some ligaments cross within a joint, such as certain ligaments of the stifle joint (the horse's equivalent of our knee joint) and are called the *cruciate ligaments*.

Composition

Ligaments are similar to tendons in composition. They consist of parallel bundles of dense connective tissue. Type I collagen, the same type that makes up tendons, primarily makes up this connective tissue.

Tendons and Ligaments of the Lower Foreleg

This is where you'll learn names of tendons and ligaments, where on the leg they start and stop and how they help the leg move.

The Superficial Digital Flexor (SDF) Tendon and the Associated Superior Check Ligament

The *superficial digital flexor (SDF)* tendon is commonly injured in the horse, especially in racing Thoroughbreds and Quarter Horses. This is one of the most extensively studied tendons. Any equine athlete is highly prone to SDF tendon injury, often called the "bowed tendon."

The SDF muscle runs along the back of the horse's *radius bone* (the large bone above the horse's knee, or *carpus*). The muscle narrows near the carpus to form the SDF tendon (see Figure 7).

The *superior (radial) check ligament* attaches the SDF muscle to the radius above the carpus. We call it a ligament even though it

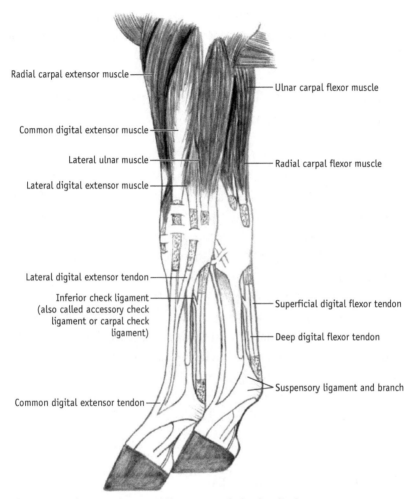

Fig. 7. Muscles, tendons and ligaments of the forelimb.

attaches a muscle to a bone (a quirk you'll have to live with). We'll discuss the *inferior* or *carpal check ligament* with the *deep digital flexor tendon*. Veterinarians believe check ligaments protect or "check" the tendon from overstretching, hence their name.

The SDF tendon, round in a cross section, passes through the carpal canal on the back of the horse's carpus. As it continues down the limb, the SDF tendon becomes flattened. It is shaped like a skinny half moon, and it cups itself over the much rounder deep *digital flexor tendon*. At the fetlock joint, the SDF tendon branches into two small tendons that attach onto the pastern bones, helping to support them.

The Deep Digital Flexor (DDF) Tendon and the Inferior Check Ligament

Injury to the *deep digital flexor (DDF)* tendon is uncommon. The DDF muscle runs along the back of the horse's radius and narrows to form the DDF tendon just above the knee. It joins the SDF tendon through the carpal canal behind the knee. The DDF tendon is round in cross section. The inferior (carpal) check ligament begins its attachment at the knee's base then descends and attaches to the DDF tendon at the mid-cannon bone.

The DDF tendon passes through a tendon sheath at the fetlock's back. Synovial fluid in the sheath provides lubrication and nutrients to the tendons. Below the fetlock, the DDF tendon widens and becomes flat, crosses the navicular bone, descends into the foot and attaches to the third *phalanx* or coffin bone. The coffin bone is encased within the hoof wall. A navicular bursa, or fluid-filled sac, lies between the DDF tendon and the navicular bone to cushion the tendon as it bends.

The Suspensory Ligament

It is common for equine athletes (especially racehorses) to injure the suspensory ligament. The Standardbred horse often injures this ligament because this breed suffers from frequent splint bone fractures. In the foreleg, the suspensory ligament originates behind the cannon bone below the knee and descends along the cannon bone and deep to the DDF tendon. The ligament divides into two branches, each of which attaches to one *sesamoid* bone. Sesamoid bones are little bones located on each side of the rear fetlock joint. The branches continue from the sesamoid bone, coursing toward the pastern's front. There, they join the *common digital extensor*

DEFINITIONS

Carpus: knee.

Radius: the large bone above the horse's knee.

Navicular bone: a small bone in the foot.

Coffin bone: the last bone in the foot, completely encased by the hoof.

Phalanxes: bones of the pastern and in the foot. (For example, the coffin bone is also called the third phalanx.)

Sesamoid bones: two small bones on each side of the rear fetlock joint.

---

tendon, a tendon on the front of the leg (see Figure 7). The suspensory ligament's primary function is to stabilize the horse's lower leg (especially the fetlock joint) and prevent its overextension.

The Sesamoidean Ligaments

Sesamoidean ligament injury is uncommon. The sesamoidean ligaments help stabilize the fetlock joint (see Figures 8 and 9). They include:

- Oblique and straight sesamoidean ligaments. These are located behind the pastern, deep under the DDF tendon.

- Intersesamoidean ligaments. These are located between the two sesamoid bones.

- Collateral sesamoidean ligaments. These are located on each side of the fetlock joint.

- Cruciate sesamoidean ligaments. These are attached at each sesamoid bone's base and cross to attach to the opposite side of the pastern.

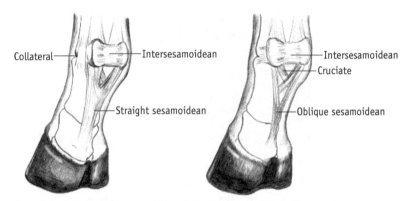

Figs. 8 and 9. Two layers of the fetlock sesamoidean ligaments.

The Palmar Anular Ligament

The *palmar anular ligament* is an inelastic band of fibrous tissue that covers the fetlock joint's back. It creates the channel through which the DDF and SDF tendons course and holds them firmly in place against the fetlock bones. Although injury to the anular ligament is uncommon, it can cause problems if there is swelling and injury to tendons that run through the channel. Palmar anular ligament problems are discussed in Chapter 3, "How and Why Injuries Occur."

The Foreleg Extensor Tendons

Extensor tendons are on the front of the horse's forelegs and assist in moving (extending) the horse's leg forward. Not only do they work with the extensor muscles (muscles that extend or move the leg forward), they also help stabilize the front joints in this region (see Figure 7).

There are three extensor tendons in the foreleg: the *extensor carpi radialis tendon*, the *common digital extensor tendon*, and the *lateral digital extensor tendon*. Each tendon has a tendon sheath where it moves over the knee joint. The last two have their own bursa sac where they traverse the fetlock joint.

The Extensor Carpi Radialis Tendon

This tendon originates from the muscle with the same name, which is located on the front of the horse's forearm above the knee. Like a large rubber band, it starts above the knee and stops and attaches on the front of the cannon bone. This tendon extends the knee joint and helps move the leg forward.

The Common Digital Extensor Tendon

This tendon originates from the common digital extensor muscle that runs next to the extensor carpi radialis muscle. However, unlike the extensor carpi radialis, this tendon descends and attaches to the horse's coffin bone. The word *digit* refers to the horse's foot. This tendon extends the horse's toe forward. Hence its name, the common *digital* extensor tendon.

The Lateral Digital Extensor Tendon

The lateral digital extensor tendon originates from the muscle with the same name. This is one of the smallest foreleg muscles. The tendon runs behind the common digital muscle/tendon unit and on the side of the leg, where it attaches on the first pastern bone just beneath the fetlock joint. It extends the horse's leg.

Tendons and Ligaments of the Lower Hind Leg

The function of tendons and ligaments of the hind leg are the same as the foreleg, although they're injured less often. They bear much less force than the foreleg due to a difference in the weight distribution. A horse's forelegs carry about 70 percent of his weight. This is the reason for the vast numbers of foreleg tendon and ligament injuries. Therapy principles are identical for the front and hind legs.

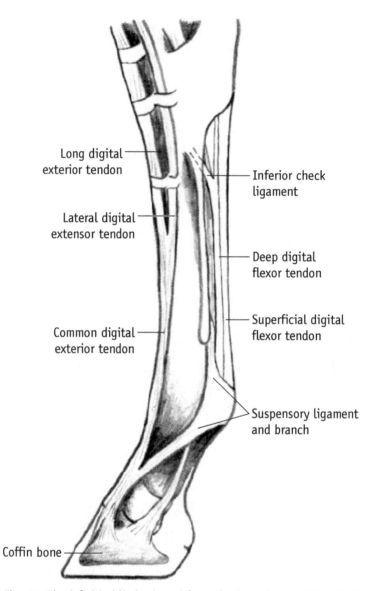

Long digital
exterior tendon

Inferior check
ligament

Lateral digital
extensor tendon

Deep digital
flexor tendon

Superficial digital
flexor tendon

Common digital
exterior tendon

Suspensory ligament
and branch

Coffin bone

Fig. 10. The left hind limb viewed from the lateral aspect (outside).

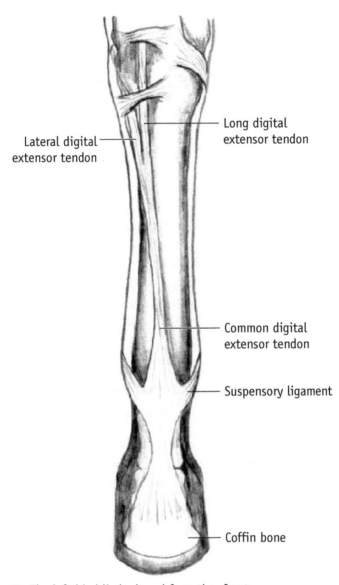

Lateral digital
extensor tendon

Long digital
extensor tendon

Common digital
extensor tendon

Suspensory ligament

Coffin bone

Fig. 11. The left hind limb viewed from the front.

Different muscles give rise to the hind legs' tendons. Although the anatomy is similar to that of the foreleg, there are some key differences (see Figures 10 and 11).

- There exist two (rather than three, as in the forelimb) primary extensor tendons: the long digital extensor tendon and the lateral digital extensor tendon.

- There is no superior check ligament of the superficial digital flexor tendon.

In Summary

Learning anatomy is fun for some, but boring or challenging for others. However, knowing anatomy is important to understanding what occurs in your horse's legs. It is easier to understand and deal with injuries if you understand how the horse's body functions.

- Tendons connect muscle to bone.

- Ligaments, in most cases, connect bone to bone.

- Tendons help legs flex and extend, and provide support and shock absorption.

- The horse's forelegs carry about 70 percent of his weight. This is why they are injured more often than the hind legs.

Chapter 3

How and Why Injuries Occur

Now that you know a little about anatomy, let's look at how and why injuries occur and learn a little terminology so you'll be able to talk with your veterinarian more effectively.

Terminology

Veterinarians and doctors love their jargon. Sometimes it's confusing to horse owners, but you need to know the terminology when you talk with your vet. It's important to understand what your vet is saying. This section focuses on accurate terminology.

Strain—Damage to a tendon caused by overuse or overstress. It can range from minor inflammation (discussed in Chapter 1, "Diagnosing Tendon and Ligament Injuries") to complete disruption or tearing of the tendon from its bony attachment (avulsion). Strains can be further classified into the following:

- *Tendinitis*—The inflammation of the tendon and tendon-muscle attachments. It refers specifically to inflammation of the flexor tendons in the horse (SDF and DDF tendons) due to excessive strain.

- *Tendosynovitis*—The inflammation of the tendon in the region associated with a tendon sheath. For example, a tendon sheath lesion in the DDF tendon where it passes over the fetlock is tendosynovitis.

- *Desmitis*—The inflammation of a ligament. For example, injury to the suspensory ligament is referred to as suspensory ligament desmitis.

- *Core lesion*—A lesion that occurs in the center of the tendon or ligament. We can detect core lesions with ultrasonography. If you took a cross section of the tissue, the core lesion looks like the hole in a doughnut. In an ultrasound, it can appear lengthwise like the center of a railroad track (without the crossing rails). The white outer "track" is the good tendon. The longer dark middle track is the lesion.

We refer to the thickening that occurs at the site of SDF tendon injury as a "bowed tendon." We also classify tendonitis or tendosynovitis according to location: high, middle or low. You may have heard of a "high bow" or a "mid-cannon bow." This refers to a horse who has strained the upper or middle portion of his superficial digital flexor tendon, respectively.

How Tendon and Ligament Injuries Occur

Now that you understand the terminology, let's look at how and why tendon and ligament injuries occur. Tendonitis or tendosynovitis (tendon injury) results from severe strain to the flexor tendons, which is associated with heavy loading (a lot of force) and overstretching the tendon. Direct trauma, such as striking the tendon with a hoof, or a tendon laceration can also cause a tendon injury (discussed later in this chapter).

The fact that racehorses and other competition horses suffer more tendon injuries than trail horses do indicates that physical

COMMON TENDON INJURIES

Tendinitis and tendosynovitis are common injuries. They occur most often in the foreleg's SDF tendon of racing Thoroughbreds and Quarter Horses, jumpers, endurance animals and barrel racers. Standardbred racehorses most often injure their suspensory ligament in the hind leg. The second most common injuries are foreleg injuries to the suspensory ligament and SDF tendons. SDF tendinitis seldom occurs in the hind leg in horses except the Standardbred. Check ligament desmitis can occur with tendinitis.

stress contributes to these injuries. Although we have little data in scientific literature indicating the exact stress on leg tendons during jumping or galloping, researchers know that normal tendon and ligament strain is in the range of 8.5 to 15 percent. This is the number that results from dividing the tendon's lengthening during weight bearing by the tendon's original length. Researchers also know that weight-bearing tendons are maximally stretched during maximal exercise, such as a Thoroughbred racehorse running at top speed. This means that there is a very low safety margin, especially in animals running at top speeds, which includes many different types of athletes in addition to racehorses.

Although the exact causes of tendon and ligament injuries aren't quite clear, most researchers agree that several factors combine to result in tendinitis or desmitis. Repetitive weakening and small amounts of damage from overstressing are more likely to cause injury than one catastrophic event. This microdamage occurs during the repetitive stretching of collagen fibers during heavy exercise. Early injury causes *edema* (swelling) between tendon fibers. If exercise continues, the blood vessels may rupture and bleed. The owner or trainer may be completely unaware of this damage.

CONTRIBUTING FACTORS TO TENDON INJURY

- Muscle fatigue from improper conditioning

- Deep ground conditions such as deep sand, mud, unevenness

- Sudden turns, especially on unconditioned limbs

- Excessive toe length, sloping pastern, improper shoeing

- Tight-fitting bandages and boots

- Lack of body coordination, as in youngsters

- Disproportionate body weight to tendon strength

- Direct trauma—striking tendon with hoof or object

Researchers have identified tendon lesions in biopsies and necropsies (autopsies) under the microscope from horses who looked clinically normal to the trainer's eye. The researchers found that the subclinically (undetectable to the eye) damaged tendons contained a type of collagen that is less mature (Type III collagen). This collagen decreases the tendon strength and predisposes the horse to an injury.

The tendon's thickness may also contribute to its degeneration. The most common site of SDF tendon injury is in the middle of the tendon, where there is the smallest cross-sectional area. Excessive load (force) per unit area on the tendon causes small tears and damage. For example, if a horse makes a hard landing and stresses a tendon at the thinnest point, it may become injured. Think of a rubber band that is worn away in one section. If you pull, it will break at that point. Thin points in tendons also have fewer blood vessels, which may make this area more susceptible to injury.

Other factors, such as muscle fatigue, may contribute to injury. Like tendons and ligaments, muscles can also function as shock absorbers. When a muscle is tired, it becomes stiff and inelastic. At this point, tendons have to absorb the shock, resulting in excessive

force being placed on them. Muscle fatigue leads to tendon and ligament overuse, which is why racehorses and other competitive
horses who are not warmed up or properly conditioned are at a high
risk for injury. If you have a competitive horse, he must be conditioned for the work. Not only will training condition his heart and
lungs, it will also build muscle strength and body coordination,
which will help prevent injury.

Other contributing factors to injury include ground conditions
(such as mud and unevenness) and sudden turns. These turns may
cause an overexertion. Abnormal fetlock angulation due to muscle
weakness or conformation, excessive pastern slope, improper shoeing and too much length in the toe may also contribute to tendon
injury. A longer toe or sloped pastern (see Figure 12) would cause
a longer time for the horse to "break over the toe" or to lift the leg
back off the ground.

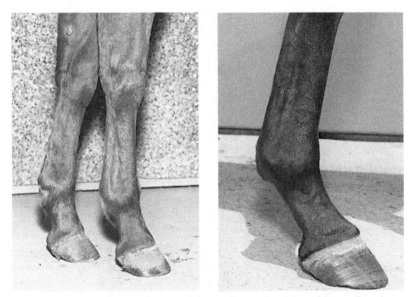

Fig. 12. On the left are short upright pasterns. Compare this to the photo
on the right that shows a long sloping pastern. Long sloping pasterns are
associated with increased tendon and ligament injury because the fetlock
hyperextends further (drops toward the ground), stretching the tendons and
ligaments.

The longer it takes for the horse to complete a full cycle of lifting his leg and putting it on the ground, the longer the fetlock is extended and pushed into the ground and the longer the tendons are stretched. Although little scientific literature supports this theory, it makes sense from a shoeing and conformation point of view.

Tight-fitting bandages and boots can also cause injury. A tight bandage or boot acts like an elastic cord that constricts the leg and can cause "bandage bow." Lack of coordination (as seen in youngsters), and disproportionate body weight to tendon strength can also cause tendon injury.

Finally, direct trauma can cause tendon and ligament injuries. Horses may strike their front tendons with a back hoof, or they may lacerate a tendon. Although both of these injuries are uncommon, they may result in severe consequences. Tendon lacerations are veterinary emergencies and require surgery (see Figure 13).

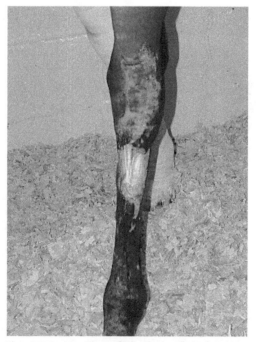

Fig. 13. Laceration of the long digital extensor tendon over the horse's rear cannon bone.

In Summary

Despite the existing research in this area, we still don't know exactly what causes tendon and ligament injuries. But we do know what factors contribute to them. Learn the jargon; knowing terminology will help you converse with your vet. You can control some risk factors for injury by making sure that:

- Your horse is properly shod and has balanced hooves.

- Your horse is well conditioned for his task and properly warmed up.

- You apply boots and bandages properly.

- You monitor the ground conditions and avoid deep mud or sand.

- Your horse's stall is free from sharp wire or objects that can cause a laceration.

Chapter 4

Treating Acute Injuries, and Directed Therapy

Healing takes time, especially with tendon and ligament injuries. Be patient because the amount of time may mean the difference between a good and a poor prognosis. Tendon and ligament injuries can be serious, and your horse's best chance at making a full recovery might depend on the amount of time you rest him. Your horse may not be fully healed for up to a year, even if he only has a moderate injury.

If time is the most important factor in recovery, the second most important factor is the right therapy at the right time. Choosing the right treatment is essential to ensuring that the injury heals properly over time. Your vet may prescribe you to do one thing for a few weeks and then something else for another few weeks. This is because the injury is going through phases of healing. For example, during the first week of recovery, your horse requires stall rest and aggressive measures to decrease inflammation. During the next four weeks, your vet may want you to start a mild exercise schedule. Your horse may have several treatments over the course of weeks or months.

Therapy is a lot like following a chocolate cake recipe. Just as not all chefs agree on the best recipe for chocolate cake but may agree on most of the basic ingredients, not all vets agree on the same treatments. However, there are basic therapies that all good veterinarians use. This chapter focuses on these basic therapies and what to do, when and why.

Let's look at how a tendon or a ligament heals so the therapies will make sense to you.

How Injuries Heal

To understand many of the therapeutic options and why they help your horse, it is important to have some idea of how tendons and ligaments heal. This will help you know why you do what and when, and how it's going to help.

Initial Injury

After injury, the body repairs the tendon or ligament as it would other tissues. In tendon injury, the tendon's tissue and blood vessels tear in the injured region. The tendon fibers disrupt and separate, a process that worsens when blood and fluid leak into the tendon. Bleeding causes a clot to form within three to four weeks. The injury also starts the initial inflammatory process which, unless it goes awry, is an important component of healing. Inflammatory cells migrate to the tendon's damaged area to clean out the damaged tissue over time. To do this, inflammatory cells secrete enzymes that break down the damaged tissue so the body can remove it from the region.

However, if the inflammation is allowed to go unchecked, the enzymes can damage good tissue, also. This is why you must reduce inflammation in tendon therapy. Inflammation can also cause the tendon to stick abnormally to surrounding tissue, which will impair tendon gliding. This is another reason why it's important to reduce inflammation.

Early Healing: From One to Six Months

New blood vessels and immature tissue replace the clot formed in the early weeks after an injury. Once inflammation has removed the dead tissue, the tendon replaces the lost tendon fibers with new ones, but they aren't as strong. These fibers are made of a weaker collagen called Type III collagen, which is very different from normal tendon fibrils. Cells called fibroblasts begin to produce the new Type III collagen, which is less mature, weaker, arranged in smaller diameter fibers and haphazardly arranged rather than arranged in parallel fibers like the normal tendon's original Type I collagen.

Remodeling: From Six Months On

The immature Type III collagen is slowly replaced with the stronger Type I collagen, but not completely. Rest, time, healing and slow return to work eventually increase the tendon fibers' diameter and strength, and reorient them in a more parallel fashion. This is why early controlled exercise is so important to the recuperating tendon. Controlled exercise will also help decrease scar tissue. More on rest schedules follows in this chapter.

Ideal healing results in a strong tendon or ligament with minimal to no scar tissue. The tendon will never be as strong as before, but your horse will regain most of its function. Although many competition horses may no longer be able to perform at their peaks, they can perform well at lower levels.

Healing, especially of tendon and ligament injuries, requires time and patience. The entire process of initial inflammation, early healing and remodeling requires from 9 to 12 months, although additional healing may occur for years. Expect up to a year for your horse to fully recover.

Therapy for Acute Injuries: The First 48 Hours to One Week

The overall goals of therapy are to reduce inflammation, to minimize scar tissue formation, and to promote healing and restoration. For the first 48 hours through a week, the therapeutic process begins with decreasing inflammation. The treatment schedule and methods follow.

Cold Therapy

Cold is highly effective in decreasing inflammation and is safe and easy to apply. Cold water hosing works well, but a colder temperature is better. Ice packs or an ice-water slurry (a mixture of water and ice) work best to get the leg cold enough to make a difference in reducing inflammation. Ice-water slurries deep-cool tissues faster than ice or cold water alone and are the best method of cold therapy. However, any cold therapy is better than none. You should apply cold in the first 48 hours to one week after injury, four times in 24 hours for no more than 30 minutes. Studies show that longer exposure to cold will cause blood vessels to dilate, which can increase swelling.

Bandaging

Bandaging applies pressure to the leg and controls swelling by pushing fluid out of the area and preventing new leakage from dilated blood vessels. Decreasing swelling is important because too much fluid or blood in the tendon further disrupts the tendon fibers and causes more damage. You can apply support bandages between each period of cold therapy. (See Figure 14 for properly applied support bandages.) Note that these bandages have adequate padding and are evenly distributed over the leg. Appropriate padding is important for any bandaged limb, since improper bandaging can cause further tendon injury.

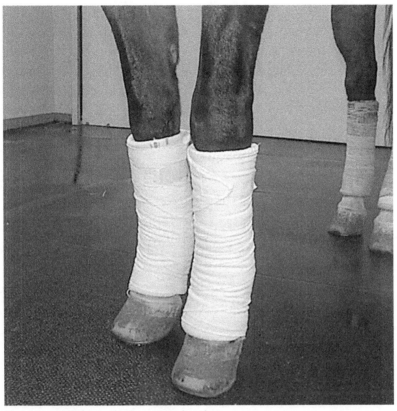

Fig. 14. Properly applied support bandages.

Nonsteroidal Anti-inflammatory Drugs (NSAIDs)

Nonsteroidal anti-inflammatory drugs such as phenylbutazone (bute) or flunixin meglumine (Banamine) administered for the first one to two weeks after a tendon or ligament injury are important to reduce inflammation, swelling and pain. Neither drug has been shown to be more beneficial than the other, although bute is less expensive. Discuss with your veterinarian which NSAID he or she prefers and why. These medications may have side effects if given long term. They are best used in the initial stages of an injury for the express purpose of decreasing inflammation.

Vets sometimes use corticosteroids injected into the tendon to decrease inflammation. These powerful drugs have multiple side effects and shouldn't be used in treating tendons. Corticosteroids are detrimental to tendon healing, resulting in delayed healing and a weaker tendon. Calcification or hardening can also occur at the injection site; this impedes the stretching capability so necessary for tendons.

Rest

Your horse should be on strict stall rest for the first 48 hours after an injury or more depending on the injury. Your veterinarian will tell you based on the nature and degree of your horse's injury how long he will need stall rest. After this, your veterinarian will most likely have you start hand walking for 10 minutes twice daily, working up to 40 minutes a day. This will continue for 60 to 90 days after the initial injury. A return-to-work schedule follows later in this chapter.

Dimethyl Sulfoxide (DMSO)

DMSO is a topical liquid medication used for its anti-inflammatory effects. It decreases inflammation and neutralizes certain molecules released from inflammatory cells. It also protects cells against free radicals, those molecules that occur from lack of blood supply that can further damage tissue. Your vet can administer DMSO intravenously or orally via a nasogastric tube. You can also apply it locally to the tendon.

DMSO is a vehicle. Therefore, vets have used it to carry corticosteroids or other substances through the skin to the tendon. It can be used under a wrap; however, it can cause blistering so it is important to start with small amounts. Most veterinarians feel it is best if used during the first week after an injury, since this is the time when inflammation control is important. No controlled studies show the effectiveness of DMSO, but it is standard therapy for many inflammatory conditions at barns all over the world. Your veterinarian can direct its use for your horse.

DEFINITION

Vehicle: a substance that carries other substances across the skin.

DMSO is very volatile. If you get it on your skin, you will absorb it. Both people and horses exposed to DMSO will smell like garlic. If you use DMSO with other medications and get those on your skin, you can carry those medications into your bloodstream, so it is important to use latex gloves when applying DMSO.

Polysulfated Glycosaminoglycan (PSGAG; Adequan)

Glycosaminoglycans (GAGs) are a component of joint cartilage. GAGs, along with other glycoproteins, occupy the spaces between the collagen fibers that make up joint cartilage. PSGAG (a special GAG containing additional sulfates) is a drug used in the treatment of joint diseases such as osteoarthritis. Vets call it a chonroprotective drug, meaning that it protects cartilage, and is used to prevent, retard or reverse the changes that occur with osteoarthritis. Humans also use PSGAG for osteoarthritis. The drug works by inhibiting enzymes associated with cartilage breakdown and reducing inflammation. It is also used to treat tendinitis. PSGAGs used in the early phase after a tendon injury may be effective in reducing pain and swelling and may improve the outcome of therapy. Some horses have returned to their previous work but, in one study, less than 50 percent of horses were able to return to racing. One study treated horses with tendon lesions with either PSGAG intramuscularly or with a control medicine for eight weeks. Those in the PSGAG-treated group were significantly improved relative to the control group's tendons, suggesting that PSGAG therapy may help tendon healing.

Your vet will administer the PSGAG either around the tendon lesion or in the muscle within 28 to 48 hours after an injury every four days up to seven doses. Discuss this therapy with your veterinarian, who will have his or her own experiences with the drug to share with you so you can make an informed decision.

Alternative Therapies

Owners and practitioners have used cold laser therapy, electrical stimulation, magnetic therapy and therapeutic ultrasound with varying results. No controlled clinical studies exist to document their effectiveness at decreasing inflammation or increasing healing rates, although many owners and trainers have used these methods and feel they achieve good results. Therapeutic ultrasound studies done on cells in tissue culture (not in the whole animal, but in a petri dish) show that this method does stimulate collagen synthesis. Therefore, there is early evidence that it may be useful in the early treatment of tendon and ligament injuries. (See more in Chapter 8.)

Directed Therapy after the First Week: Guiding the Repair Process

Keeping inflammation in check during this healing phase is still important. Your horse will most likely still be getting NSAIDs and should be wearing support bandages. Controlled exercise is critical. (A sample schedule follows.) Some medications injected into the tendon show some promise in helping the repair process.

Controlled Exercise

Once the initial 48 hours to one week have passed and you get the go-ahead from your veterinarian, you can start walking your horse for 10 minutes twice daily, working up to 40 minutes a day depending on his lesion. Discuss a schedule first with your veterinarian.

Walking will continue for 60 to 90 days after the initial injury, depending on your horse's progress. He should not have access to unrestricted exercise such as pasture or arena turnout during the first four to six months because the injured tendon or ligament cannot withstand sudden force such as jumping around; the horse is highly susceptible to reinjury during this time. Consult with your veterinarian regarding exercise. This exercise chart is only an example and your vet should approve any and all exercise. Each injury will require a unique exercise chart.

This chart represents an example of a controlled exercise program. The severity of the injury may dictate that the exercise program be altered. For example, a horse with a very severe injury may continue to walk during the 60- to 90-day period, whereas in mild cases the horse can either be trotted for 5 minutes or be ridden at

Sample Exercise Chart

Days after Injury	Exercise Type and Duration
0–30 days	Handwalking, 10 min twice daily
30–60 days	Handwalking, increasing slowly to 30–40 min daily
60–90 days	Trot/jog, 5 min
90–150 days	Trot/jog, 10–15 min
150–210 days	Trot/jog, 20–25 min
210–240 days	Canter, 5 min/gallop 1 mile every other day (racehorse)
240–270 days	Canter 10 min/gallop 1 mile every day (racehorse)
270–300 days	Low jumping/short breeze (racehorse)
300–330 days	Normal jumping/breezes (racehorse)
330–360 days	Competition

Chart adapted with permission from Mary Beth Whitcomb, DVM, University of California-Davis, School of Veterinary Medicine, Davis, CA.

the walk for 20 to 30 minutes. Discuss the exercise regimen with your veterinarian; it is important that the program is based on ultrasonigraphic examination of the tendon or ligament injury. It is meant to be a dynamic program, one that is altered based on new information from ultrasonigraphic examination every 90 days.

Historically, people would simply "naturally" heal their horse by turning him out to pasture and essentially forgetting about him for the next year. Research now shows that this is not wise if you wish your horse to return to work. Many horses turned out to pasture don't heal because of continual reinjury due to unrestricted exercise. In one study, 20 out of 28 Thoroughbred racehorses (71 percent) with bowed tendons that were put on a controlled exercise program returned to work at or above their previous level compared to two out of 16 (12.5 percent) that were turned out to pasture to "heal." Although this study had a very small sample, it suggests that a controlled exercise rehabilitation program is required if you want your horse to return to competition or work.

Ultrasound Exams

Your vet should perform ultrasound exams every 60 to 90 days to monitor healing progress and to prevent reinjury. Ultrasound can detect signs of tendon or ligament damage *before* a new injury occurs. With ultrasound, your veterinarian can make decisions regarding the appropriate level of exercise and whether your horse should stay at his current level or move up. Horses should not move to the next level without an ultrasound exam (see Figures 15 and 16).

Injuries of the suspensory ligament and DDF tendon tend to heal more slowly, as evidenced in Figures 17 and 18. Although there is some evidence of healing, the horse in the illustrations has a persistent lesion of his suspensory ligament after four months of rest. In this case, it may be possible to slowly progress his rehabilitation as long as the horse is not showing signs of reinjury or lameness. Discuss this with your veterinarian.

SDF tendon lesion
cross section

SDF tendon lesion
longitudinal section

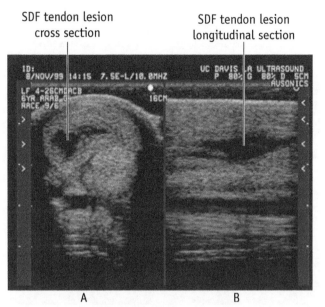

A   B

Fig. 15. Severe tear of the SDF tendon. The arrow in (A) denotes a darker circle within the gray SDF tendon. Note the normal gray DDF tendon directly beneath the SDF tendon. (B) depicts the longitudinal tendon. Note the darker band indicating a lesion in the SDF tendon at the arrow and the whiter longitudinal fibers of the normal DDF tendon underneath.

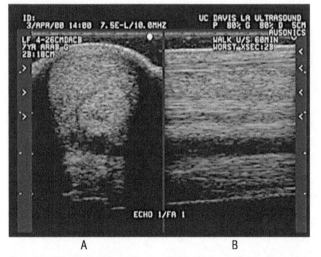

A   B

Fig. 16. Same tendon five months later. Note that the lesion is filled in and less black (A). Also note the linear arrangement of fibers in the longitudinal section (B). The tendon is markedly improved.

Suspensory ligament lesion   Same in
in cross section   longitudinal section

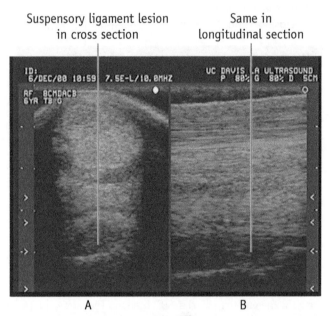

A   B

Fig. 17. Severe suspensory ligament injury. Note the black area indicating a lesion in the suspensory ligament in both (A) cross and (B) longitudinal sections.

Suspensory ligament lesion   Same in
in cross section   longitudinal section

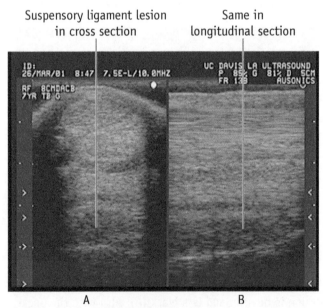

A   B

Fig. 18. Same suspensory ligament four months later. Slow progression of healing is noted.

Continued Bandaging

Even though the critical inflammatory period is quickly passing, it is important to keep the leg from swelling, or, if swollen, to get the fluid out. Once the inflammatory process is over (no less than one week), you may use heat to help dilate blood vessels, increase circulation and remove fluid. Some veterinarians and trainers use alternating cycles of hot and cold therapy to encourage fluid removal. However, no clinical studies show that this actually works. Many veterinarians advocate sweat wraps. You apply medication to the horse's leg, followed by a sheet of plastic wrap, and then bandage the leg. No studies have shown its effectiveness, but sweat wraps are commonly used; training barns use them often. Note that sweat wraps are not used in the first week after an injury when the goal is to decrease inflammation by cooling the leg, not heating it with a sweat wrap. If you don't use sweat wraps, you still need to use regular pressure bandages until swelling is no longer a problem.

Liniments and Poultices

Every training barn in the country seems to have its own formula for a special concoction used to stimulate heat and increase circulation when applied to injured legs. There is plenty of anecdotal evidence that, in many cases, liniments and poultices help draw fluid from the limb and decrease swelling. However, their effectiveness has never been studied.

Hyaluronic Acid (HA)

Hyaluronic acid (HA) is a natural substance occurring in high amounts in joints and tendon sheaths. Some veterinarians inject HA around the tendon lesion to promote healing. However, evidence for the use of HA to treat tendon and ligament injuries is controversial. One study in which researchers injected HA into the tendon lesion, then followed the horse's lesion with ultrasound and clinical examination, suggested that almost 78 percent recovered, 12 percent improved, about 5 percent were unsuccessful and 5 percent had rein-jury. Although the authors of the study concluded that they had a successful therapy that may be superior to conventional therapy, their data does not demonstrate the efficacy of the drug. We don't know if the 78 percent would have improved without the HA. Another study looking at the use of HA on tendon injuries compared to controls showed no difference in outcomes. However, there were trends toward less lameness in HA-treated tendons and better heal-ing on ultrasound examination relative to control tendons. It appears that HA injections may help, but more studies are needed. HA has also been used to help suspensory ligament desmitis.

Beta-aminoproprionitrile Fumarate (BAPN; Bapten)

Beta-aminoproprionitrile fumarate (Bapten) inhibits an enzyme responsible for collagen cross-linking in early tendon repair. During early healing, the body arranges the collagen fibers haphazardly, but a linear arrangement is desirable. Bapten encourages a more linear fiber pattern by decreasing early collagen cross-linking in the ten-don. It decreases the rate of reinjury but doesn't speed healing. It is best injected in the tendon lesion for five treatments total, adminis-tered two to three days apart. The ideal time to start therapy is 30 to 60 days after the initial injury, when the cross-linking enzyme is most active. Note that no studies have yet addressed the long-term effects of decreasing cross-linking. As of this writing, this drug is off the market because the expense (involving five vet visits) and length of treatment (up to a year) kept it from becoming popular with horse owners. However, those issues may be solved in the future and the drug may become available again.

Old-Time Remedies: What Not to Do

Blistering and pin-firing are two methods that have been in use for over a hundred years; many old-time veterinarians used them to treat tendon and ligament injuries. Unfortunately, some vets still use these methods, but their use constitutes animal abuse.

Blistering refers to the application of caustic solutions, such as phenol or red mercury, to the region of injury. The agent causes significant irritation, leading to swelling and sloughing of the skin. Proponents say that blistering increases circulation. There is no evidence whatsoever that blistering increases circulation to the underlying tendons. The horse is in severe pain and very lame during this time, requiring complete stall rest, the only benefit to blistering. Discuss all other therapeutic options with your veterinarian and choose a regime that fits with the equine veterinary industry standards. If your veterinarian wants to blister your horse, find a new vet.

Pin-firing is another outdated and ineffective therapy for tendon and ligament injures. A hot iron in the shape of the tip of a pen is pressed into the horse's skin, burning holes through to the underlying tendon or ligament. Old timers will claim that the procedure releases fluid and creates a tough, and therefore supporting, scar around the tendon that may protect it from future injury. Research demonstrates that firing does *nothing* to promote circulation or to help a horse's tendon or ligament injury. It does form a scar, like any wound. Firing your horse will cause him tremendous pain and enforce rest, similar to blistering.

Again, if your vet wants to use firing on your horse, find another vet. Choose a veterinarian who follows the veterinary literature and attends continuing education conferences. You want a vet who can communicate modern ideas about the care and treatment of your horse, and who will help your horse rehabilitate according to industry-standard rehabilitation schedules with modern medicine. This is what you would expect and deserve from your medical doctor, and it is what you should expect from your veterinarian.

Prognosis

Although the proper rehabilitation process is tedious and long, it will give your horse a chance to return successfully to showing, racing, jumping or any other athletic event. However, your horse's prognosis depends on the structure damaged and the severity and degree of the original lesion. For example, a 20 percent tear of the DDF tendon has a much worse prognosis than a 20 percent tear of the SDF tendon. Your horse's job also plays a role. A racehorse with a 30 percent tear of his SDF tendon might not be able to race again, but could become a successful hunter or pleasure animal. On the other hand, a child's pony used for trail riding with the same injury will likely be able to stay in his current job.

The most important factors in your horse's prognosis are the compliance of you and your horse. The rehabilitation program takes commitment, patience and time. Many fit horses are difficult to work with when suddenly confined and not on their usual exercise program. It is critical to work with your veterinarian to come up with a plan that works for your situation. It is this plan that will help ensure that your horse has the best chance to return to his prior level of performance (see Figures 19 and 20).

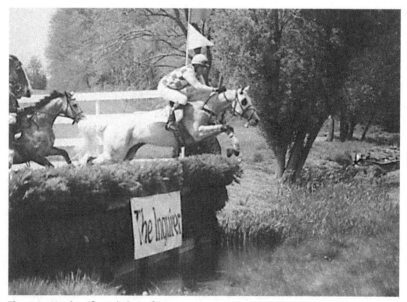

Fig. 19. Having fun, injury free.

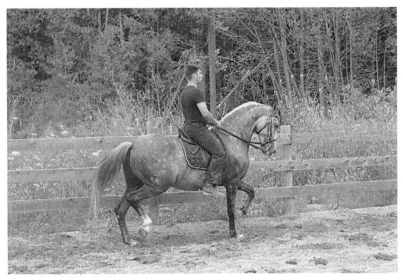

Fig. 20. Back to work.

In Summary

- Healing takes time. Your compliance and patience are the best predictors for success.

- Tendon and ligament injuries heal in stages. Knowing these stages helps you understand your veterinarian's treatment plan.

- Decreasing inflammation is one of the most important aspects of initial therapy.

- Controlled exercise is important to proper tendon and ligament healing.

- Many drugs are available to assist healing. Talk to your veterinarian about which ones might be best for your horse's injury.

- Know what treatment options are part of modern medicine and what are part of the past. Never blister or pin-fire your horse.

- A good working relationship with your veterinarian and your compliance with his or her treatment plan presents the greatest chance for success.

Chapter 5

Surgical Therapies

Although medical management of tendon and ligament injuries is the mainstay of therapy, certain surgical options may be valuable in treating some injuries. This chapter covers surgical techniques that may be appropriate, depending on your horse's injuries. They include tendon splitting, superior check ligament desmotomy, annular ligament desmotomy and surgical repair of lacerations.

Tendon lacerations are difficult to treat overall and require the owner's time and commitment to heal properly. Depending on the tendon, your horse may be able to return to work or may end up becoming a trail horse. Check your horse's living quarters—whether a box stall, paddock or pasture—for anything that could possibly result in a tendon injury and remove it. Of course, if your horse lives with his buddies in a pasture, you can never stop the occasional kick that could end in a tendon laceration. In that case, it is best to hope that it is an extensor tendon, not one of the flexors.

Tendon Splitting

Tendon splitting is a technique used to remove the blood and fluid from the core lesion of the tendon. Its popularity changes, but it has come back into favor and many veterinary referral hospitals as well as field veterinarians use the procedure.

Tendon splitting was used first in 1964 to promote formation of new blood vessels, thus helping healing. Then in the late 1960s and early 1970s the procedure went out of favor because studies showed that splitting healthy tendons diminished blood flow. However, studies in the 1990s confirm that tendon splitting in the first few days following an injury decreases the lesion size and promotes healing. One study showed a 44 percent reduction in lesion size and severity following injury after the tenth day. They also established that 81 percent of the horses were able to return to work and 68 percent competed at the same level as they had prior to injury. This study was impressive because the lesions described were high grade (severe) and encompassed up to 80 percent of the cross-sectional area of the tendon.

Researchers believe that splitting creates a communication between the tendon core and the surrounding tissue that promotes faster repair of blood flow and collagen production and decreases inflammatory edema more rapidly.

The procedure is simple: the horse is sedated but remains standing, and the affected leg is treated with local anesthesia. An ultrasound exam must be performed prior to the procedure to locate the lesion. After the local anesthesia is administered, the veterinarian stabs a scalpel or a large bore needle through the tendon's side, directly into the core lesion. Some veterinarians fan the blade up and down. They should not cut into healthy tendon. The scalpel blade is placed parallel to the fibers so that it does not cut fibers crossways. This releases fluid from the core lesion, similiar to popping a water balloon.

A vet should only perform this procedure in an injury's early phase (usually within the first week or two after the horse is injured), when there is a fluid-filled core lesion. After the first few weeks, a clot (which tendon splitting cannot remove) will form.

Superior Check Ligament Desmotomy

In 1986, superior check ligament desmotomy (cutting of a ligament) was first described and proposed as a novel therapy for SDF tendon injuries. The superior check ligament originates on the back of the horse's radius (forearm bone) and descends to connect to the SDF tendon. It "checks" (or restricts) the length that the SDF tendon can stretch. It is believed that cutting the superior check ligament will cause the SDF tendon to lengthen. As a result, the muscle will absorb more of the load and the entire unit will stretch more, thus protecting the SDF tendon. Studies indicate that this may be true.

In one study of 62 Thoroughbreds, 92 percent of the horses were able to train and race after surgery, 66 percent started at least five races after surgery, and 48 percent maintained or increased their average earnings, while only 19 percent reinjured the tendon. These results compared favorably with another study in which 71 percent (97 of 137 horses) raced and 51 percent (70 horses) had more than five starts after surgery, although average earnings decreased in 58 percent of the horses. In another study addressing the long-term effects of check ligament desmotomy, the authors found no benefit of the surgery to decrease reinjury.

Results for superior check desmotomy are much better in the Standardbred than in the Thoroughbred racehorse. In one study of 38 horses, 92 percent (35 horses) raced after surgery and 87 percent (33 horses) started more than five races. Other studies involving this breed compare favorably. There are no other controlled studies in other breeds or in horses used for other events, such as hunters, jumpers, dressage horses or event horses, although one researcher claims that prognosis for these animals lies somewhere between that for Thoroughbreds and for Standardbreds.

As with all therapeutic options, no one treatment is a panacea that will be the best for your horse. Each animal and every injury is different. Discuss with your veterinarian or specialist what is right for your horse.

Annular Ligament Desmotomy (ALD)

The annular ligament is a tough band around the back of the fetlock that helps hold the tendons in place. Because it doesn't expand much, it can trap or constrict swollen and inflamed flexor tendons that run through it. This can worsen the tenosynovitis, resulting in pain and persistent lameness. Under certain conditions, the annular ligament may need to be cut in order to release the pressure over the flexor tendons.

Not all problems with the annular ligament are secondary to tendon injury. Annular ligament desmitis rarely occurs, but we don't understand why. When an injury occurs, the flexor tendon sheath fills with fluid above the annular ligament, which looks like a windpuff. The fetlock's back will appear uneven where the annular ligament constricts the tendon sheath.

It doesn't matter whether the primary problem is the annular ligament or a tendon injury; annular ligament constriction that impairs tendon movement is an indication for ALD. A study at Colorado State University reported that 87 percent (21 out of 24) of horses with primary annular ligament desmitis that underwent ALD became sound and 13 percent (3) improved. Fifteen other horses had tendinitis in addition to annular ligament desmitis and underwent ALD surgery. Of those horses, 38 percent (5) became sound, 54 percent (7) improved and 8 percent (1) did not improve from ALD surgery. Studies indicate that there is a more favorable outcome if the annular ligament constriction is not accompanied by extensive damage to the tendon.

Vets usually perform annular ligament desmotomy with the horse standing under local anesthetic and slight sedation. However, your vet may use general anesthesia when there is extensive tendon sheath involvement and scar tissue. The annular ligament is cut directly behind the fetlock, which relieves constriction. Typically, horses can return to full work within a few months, depending on whether there is tendon damage and to what extent the tendon sheath is involved in this damage.

Surgical Repair of Lacerations

Tendon lacerations, especially of the extensor tendons, are more common than once thought. In the foreleg, the common and lateral digital extensors are most often cut. In the hind leg, it is the long digital extensor (see Figure 21). One study showed that 89 percent

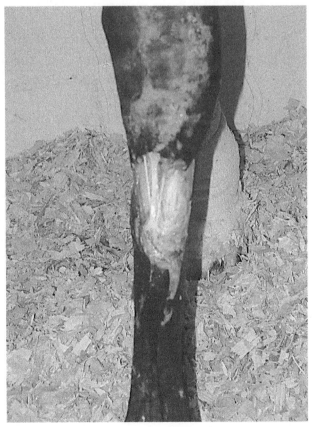

Fig. 21. Long digital extensor tendon laceration.

of lacerations involved the hind legs, making this much more common in the hind legs than the forelegs. Laceration of the flexor tendons most often occurs between the knee and the fetlock in the foreleg or the hock and the fetlock in the hind leg.

The quickest way to determine if your horse has cut a tendon without actually examining the wound is to observe his stance. Most horses with tendon lacerations will have an altered stance. A severed common digital or long digital extensor tendon will make your horse unable to extend his toe properly; he may drag the toe or "knuckle over." Typically, a horse with a severed lateral digital extensor tendon in his front or hind leg will not have a gait abnormality. A horse with flexor tendon lacerations will have a dropped fetlock and his toe may even tip up if he has lacerated both the DDF and the SDF tendons. Your vet can examine the cut after applying local anesthesia to the horse's leg.

Once your vet repairs an extensor tendon laceration, your horse has a good prognosis for a complete recovery, although it may take more than six months. Your veterinarian will thoroughly clean the region, cut away any damaged tissue and suture the tendon ends together if there is minimal contamination. In cases with a lot of dirt and debris in the wound, your veterinarian may not suture the tendon but allow it to heal by what veterinarian's call "second intention"—healing on its own without suturing. Your vet will use a cast or splint bandage to immobilize the leg following surgery. He will remove the cast after about two weeks and apply a bandage splint for an additional two weeks to prevent the fetlock from knuckling. Sometimes a horse requires a splint bandage and corrective shoeing with an extended toe instead of a cast. The treatment depends on the cut's location and severity.

Unfortunately, flexor tendon lacerations don't have as good a prognosis as extensor tendon lacerations. If both the DDF and SDF tendons are cut, your vet will usually recommend euthanasia unless the horse is very valuable and can be used as a breeding animal. However, the prognosis is poor whether the horse is an expensive Thoroughbred or a backyard pony.

If only one flexor tendon is cut, the prognosis is a bit better. Depending on the location and extent of the laceration, your veterinarian may or may not suture the tendon ends back together. Regardless, the leg must be kept immobilized with a cast or a splint bandage in order for it to heal properly. This not only prevents tension on the cut ends, but also helps establish new blood vessels. After six weeks, the veterinarian will remove the cast and apply a special shoe. He may also recommend applying passive motion, or controlled non-weight-bearing movement, to the leg to decrease scar tissue and increase the range of motion.

The prognosis for return to full athletic function after flexor tendon lacerations is poor. One study showed that 60 percent of horses with flexor tendon lacerations returned to riding soundness, but not athletic function. In another study of 50 horses, 82 percent (32 horses) were sound for riding and many returned to their intended use. However, the prognosis relies on how much damage was done to the tendon, how much time passed before the owner sought veterinary care, the amount of contamination and whether one or two tendons were cut.

The prognosis goes down if a tendon sheath is involved in the laceration. Tendon sheaths become infected easily and are difficult to treat. These injuries often result in severe lameness regardless of therapy. Tendon sheath wounds need aggressive therapy with antibiotics and possibly surgical intervention to rinse the affected area. If there's an infection, long-term therapy can be frustrating and unrewarding. It can take several months to heal chronic tendon sheath infections. Adhesions and scar tissue that form may restrict tendon movement, resulting in ongoing lameness even if treatment cured the original infection. Discuss the options with your veterinarian and decide together what the best course of action is. It's a difficult decision to put an animal down based on its poor prognosis.

In Summary

- Certain surgical therapies may be warranted for your horse's injured tendon or ligament.

- Tendon lacerations are more common than once thought.

- Tendon lacerations of the hind legs are more common than tendon lacerations of the front legs.

- Lacerations can take more than six months to heal and can be quite serious.

Chapter 6

Support Wraps, Boots and Bandages

Owners and trainers use support wraps, boots and bandages to control swelling, to give support and to provide protection. For example, show and racehorses hauled in a trailer will wear shipping boots or thick support bandages. Many trainers routinely use support wraps on their horses overnight. Boots such as skid boots, tendon guards and bell boots are used on horses performing many athletic functions, including jumping, reining, roping, team penning and dressage. While wraps and boots are useful in certain circumstances, these protective devices can turn into hazards. In this chapter, we will discuss the benefits and drawbacks of wraps and boots.

Swelling

Trainers and owners often use wraps and boots to prevent swelling. Properly applied bandages help control swelling by applying pressure to the leg. The pressure helps force fluid out of the area and keeps more fluid from leaking into the area. Pressure bandages are a necessity in tendon and ligament injuries, as discussed in Chapter 4.

Protection

Trainers and owners often use wraps and boots to protect the horse's legs. Boots and bandages afford some degree of protection, especially during exercise. Trauma can be self-induced if, for example, your horse strikes his foreleg with his hind leg during exercise or if he orreaches with his hind foot and clips the heel's coronary band (the soft tissue at the interface of the hoof and the ankle, or *pastern,* of a front foot). A horse may be prone to interfering or hitting one leg with the opposite leg. Although there are many different types of boots that provide protection from these various injuries, it's important to know that boots cannot prevent all injuries. Fast-moving legs with metal shoes attached can inflict serious damage to tendons and ligaments if struck with enough force at high speeds. Sometimes major trauma can occur despite protective boots.

You must remember that fitting the boot properly is critical. An ill-fitting boot or one that you don't put on correctly can result in more damage than no boot at all. Ask questions when you purchase the boots, or have an experienced user show you the proper way for your horse to wear them. There's nothing worse than a huge raw spot or, worse, injury from a boot that is intended to protect your horse (see Figure 22).

Support

Boots and bandages also provide support to the equine limb. Theoretically, a bandage that can increase support to the horse's leg should prevent or decrease hyperextension or dropping of the fetlock joint.

Although information on this topic is limited, studies show that certain support boots can increase the energy absorption capacity by as much as 20 percent, which could make the difference between a sound horse and an injured horse. However, this has not been

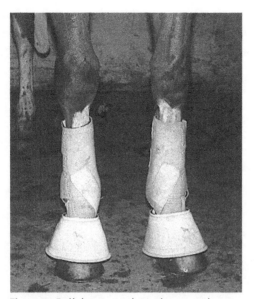

Fig. 22. Bell boots and tendon guards protect tendons and ligaments from forging
injuries.

proven through any clinical trials. When applied correctly, the
newer support bandages such as Powerflex, Leva Wrap and 3M's
Equisport bandages absorb some of the shock at slower speeds and
reduce lower leg "wobble" by restricting normal fetlock side-to-side
movement at the gallop.

Proper application is critical if support bandages are to work properly. You must wrap the bandage so the lower portion extends below
the horse's fetlock joint. If you only wrap in the cannon bone region,
the fetlock will not be supported. Various wrapping patterns (such as
figure-8 under the fetlock) offer more support than standard one-
direction wraps. Although most people think that the direction of a
wrap should always be from the front to the back, the support is the
same regardless of which way around the limb the leg is wrapped. The
key, again, is that the bandage must be wrapped below the fetlock and
that figure-8 wrapping patterns are best.

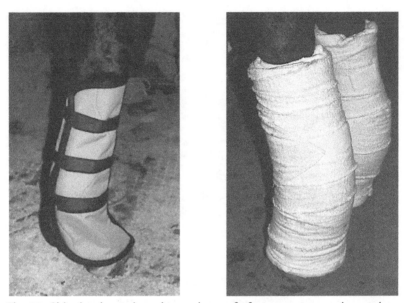

Fig. 23. Shipping boots keep horses legs safe from puncture and scratches. This horse's legs are well wrapped for protection while traveling.

Support wraps help reduce the fetlock joint's hyperextension and protect against fatigue. Companies that develop these wraps use high-speed treadmill and video equipment in bandage development research to measure the relative support obtained from varying materials and wrapping methods. Improved fastening and securing methods such as using Velcro tabs makes these newer bandages easy and quick to apply and remove. Elastic, cohesive bandages such as the three mentioned previously adhere only to themselves rather than to the horse. This eliminates the hassle and potential discomfort to the horse that may occur when adhesive bandages are removed. However, wrapping any bandage too tight can cause disaster. Apply the bandages under the guidance of experienced users so you can get the feel of what is tight enough and what is too tight for your horse.

The Biggest Problems with Boots and Bandages

Although we use boots and bandages on horses, surprisingly little is known about their beneficial or harmful effects. However, we do know that wrapping a bandage too tightly is very bad for your horse because it will constrict blood circulation to the underlying skin and leg. One result of this is a "bandage bow," a condition that damages the tendon. While this damage may not be severe, it will still take more than a few weeks to heal.

Besides applying a bandage too tightly, certain locations are inherently problematic when bandaged and can result in pressure sores. Bandaging a knee can cause pressure sores at the back over the large accessory carpal bone, a bone that pokes out backward from the knee right under the skin. Sores can develop over the point of the hock as well. Veterinarians use special wrapping techniques and methods to relieve tension over these areas that can help prevent such sores.

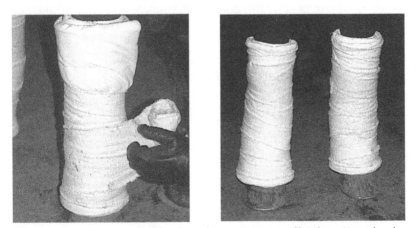

Fig. 24. Shipping wraps; side view shows proper application. May also be used as pressure wraps.

Boots and bandages have been around for many years, despite little proof that they are effective in protecting and supporting a horse's legs. However, available research does indicate that support wraps help support the fetlock joint if applied properly in horses undergoing events that require heavy strain. Any horse owner knows that boots help protect legs from opposing leg strikes or heel scrapes. However, not all boots are the same and the quality of the boot determines its effectiveness. Evaluate the work your horse is doing and make an informed decision about the best type of protection for his legs and which boot is best. Research takes time, but it is well worth it. After all, if you have a quality animal, shouldn't a quality boot go on his legs?

In Summary

- Owners and trainers use support wraps, boots and bandages to control swelling, for support and for protection.

- Although they are made to protect and support, these items can cause harm if used incorrectly.

- Apply support wraps, boots and bandages under the guidance of experienced users.

Chapter 7

Horseshoeing

Good horseshoeing is not only a science, but it is also an art. A farrier must assess the balance of the foot, whether it is flat and level, and must make corrections. There are four places a farrier looks for proper balance: from toe to heel, from side to side (medial to lateral), pastern alignment with the front of the hoof wall (hoof angle) and dynamic balance (foot placement on the ground). The farrier also assesses the length, levelness, sole, frog and foot shape and the symmetry of foot pairs before even touching a horse's foot with his blade.

Over the years, farriers, veterinarians, owners and trainers have paid attention to how the foot, and specifically the hoof angle, affects the horse's joints, tendons and ligaments. Unfortunately, there isn't much clinical data to support long-held notions. There are some studies available, but the information is not always what many in the horse world believe.

To begin understanding the role of the hoof in tendon and ligament injuries and recovery, you must first understand what a normal hoof is.

The Normal Hoof

As with the anatomy of the leg, knowing the normal foot is critical if you are to understand what can go wrong and how it will affect other structures in the leg. People within the horse industry constantly argue over the hoof angle. The hoof wall at the toe forms an angle relative to the flat ground that you can measure with a hoof angle gauge called a hoof protractor. The units of measurement for this angle are degrees. For years, many textbooks cited the normal hoof angle to be 45 to 50° for a typical horse's forefoot and 50 to 55° for a hind foot. However, farriers have observed that normal foreleg hoof angles range from 53 to 58° and hind leg hoof angles range from 55 to 60°. Researchers confirmed these observations in a study in which the average front foot hoof angle was 53.8° and the average hind leg hoof angle was 54.8°. Studies aside, it is most important that you know that each horse has his own ideal hoof angle. The angle is correct when the hoof wall and pastern are in alignment (see sidebar).

A high hoof angle refers to a heel that is too high, which will cause the line to break forward. A horse with a high hoof angle and short toe will have a clubfoot appearance. A low hoof angle refers to a heel that is too low, causing the line to break backward and resulting in hyperextension of the fetlock joint (dropping toward the ground).

HOOF ANGLES

- Correct hoof angle: Your horse's hoof angle is correct when the front wall of his hoof and pastern are in alignment. The alignment is proper when an imaginary line passed down the center of the long pastern bone is parallel to the front of the hoof wall (see Figure 25).

- High hoof angle: the heel is too high.

- Low hoof angle: the heel is too low.

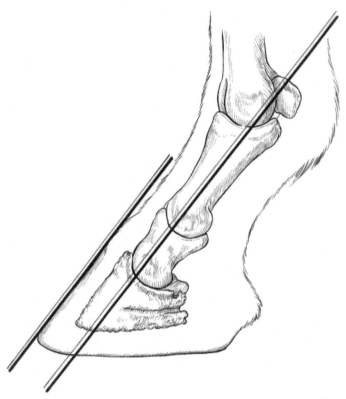

Fig. 25. A proper hoof angle. The hoof and pastern are in alignment. An imaginary line passed down the center of the long pastern bone is parallel to the front of the hoof wall.

The Effects of Horseshoeing on Tendons and Ligaments: Facts and Fallacies

It seems intuitive that alterations in the hoof angle must do something to the legs, and especially to the tendons and ligaments. Most people believe that a high hoof angle, or a raised heel, will relieve stress on the flexor tendons and ligaments. They also believe that a low hoof angle, or low heel, will strain flexor tendons because the fetlock will be hyperextended (dropping of fetlock), increasing the amount of stretch in the flexor tendons. This belief is why farriers will raise the heel with wedge pads in a horse with a flexor tendon injury. However, research shows that these beliefs aren't entirely true.

Studies show that increasing the hoof angle (raising the heel) will decrease the strain on the DDF tendon, but not on the SDF tendon or suspensory ligament. However, extremely high hoof angles (60° or more) cause extreme coffin joint flexion (the bone in the hoof) and a clubfoot appearance. Researchers have documented many problems associated with high hoof angle including coffin joint arthritis, arthritis of the extensor process (the part of the coffin bone where the common digital extensor tendon attaches), pedal osteitis (inflammation of the foot) and *increased* strain on the SDF tendon and suspensory ligament. Another study in ponies confirmed this finding.

We know that horses with low, underrun heels have more foot lameness than those with a normal hoof angle. However, researchers have not documented that an altered hoof angle contributes to more tendon or ligament injuries relative to a normal foot angle.

HIGH HOOF ANGLE PROBLEMS

Problems caused by high hoof angles include:

- Coffin joint arthritis: inflammation of the joint between the last bone and the first pastern bone

- Extensor process arthritis: arthritis of the part of the coffin bone where the extensor tendon attaches

- Pedal osteitis: inflammation of the coffin bone (a bone in the foot)

Based on the available data, researchers don't know yet whether altering the hoof angle will help a horse with a tendon or ligament injury. The once commonly held belief that raising the heel might help alleviate strain in a SDF tendon or suspensory ligament injury may actually cause the problem to get worse, according to current research. Therefore, it is important to make an informed decision with your veterinarian and farrier after discussing all of the availabe options and the reasoning behind each treatment. You will never go wrong by making sure your horse's foot is balanced with a correct hoof angle and proper toe length.

In Summary

- A balanced foot is the most important aspect of proper shoeing.

- Your horse's hoof angle is correct when the front wall of his hoof and pastern are in alignment. The alignment is proper when an imaginary line passed down the center of the long pastern bone is parallel to the front of the hoof wall.

- Not all commonly held beliefs about hoof angle are correct.

- You will never go wrong by making sure your horse's foot is balanced with a correct hoof angle and proper toe length.

Chapter 8

Alternative Therapies

Alternative therapies are treatments the conventional medical community doesn't normally use. Although these nontraditional therapies are often controversial, sometimes they do become part of mainstream therapies. For example, human chiropractic care once was considered highly "alternative" but has now gained acceptance in the mainstream and even among many physicians. This chapter presents some common alternative therapies for equine tendon and ligament injuries and presents the *scientific* research that is available for evaluating the method.

Although most of these methods have little scientific support for efficacy, many of them are considered harmless. For the horse owner who absolutely must do everything for his or her animal, some of these methods may be desirable. However, there is evidence suggesting that some may be harmful by delaying healing and, therefore, should be avoided.

Veterinary medicine is severely limited in its ability to treat equine tendon and ligament injuries, despite the substantial research that has been done in this area. The amount of time and effort that is required in treating these injuries is frustrating, and it is natural to want to do all you can to assist the process. In this case, some alternative therapies may be beneficial. It is important to understand that the number of controlled studies that have been

---

SOURCES FOR VETERINARY HOSPITALS AND VETERINARY SPECIALTY SERVICES

- For schools and for information on veterinary services and care for all animals, including horses, go to http://netvet.wustl.edu/.
- For all veterinary schools on the planet, go to http://netvet.wustl.edu/vetmed.htm.

---

conducted using these methods is few and that some alternative medicine may be harmful. Keep this in mind when deciding to treat your horse. Check out the manufacturer's claims and discuss these with your veterinarian. If you're not sure, call one of the 27 large animal referral hospitals at veterinary schools around the country and ask to speak with a specialist in equine surgery. The equine surgeons who specialize in orthopedic and soft tissue injuries will have the most up-to-date information.

Acupuncture

Veterinarians worldwide are practicing the art and science of acupuncture, a treatment approach that entails insertion of sterile needles into precise locations to stimulate repair in the body. It originated in China and has gained ground in the United States over the past 20 years. The purpose of this section is to give you a flavor for the practice, not to be an authoritative guide. I urge you to seek out information on your own, educate yourself and then proceed under the direction of your veterinarian or another veterinary professional. Additional resources are included at the end of this section.

Veterinary acupuncture in the equine industry has received more attention in the press in recent years, spurring the interest of both the public and the veterinary medical community. Increased awareness about veterinary acupuncture leads to increased research and thus a better understanding of the physiologic basis and the practical applications of acupuncture. Veterinarian acupuncturists take extensive courses and training to receive certification in this science. They are required to fulfill continuing education programs to keep them abreast of new information from year to year.

Lameness diagnosis and treatment is one of the main applications in which acupuncture is used in equine practice. It can be used as both an adjunct to the traditional lameness examination as well as an addition to the treatment of specific lameness conditions. Although it is mostly used to treat compensatory, or secondary, body pain resulting from tendon and ligament injuries rather than the primary injury, it can also be used to help diagnose why a horse may have been predisposed to injure a particular tendon or ligament.

Acupuncture points are areas on the skin of decreased electrical resistance or increased electrical conductivity. Acupuncture stimulates sensory nerves, transmitting the signal through the central nervous system to the brain. Various transmitters and hormones are then released from the brain to have their effects felt throughout the body. Acupuncture has many physiologic effects on all systems throughout the body; one mechanism cannot explain all the physiologic effects observed.

Techniques

There are numerous techniques available to stimulate acupuncture points, including dry needle stimulation, electroacupuncture (using electricity), aquapuncture (using water), acupressure and others (see Figure 26). Your veterinary acupuncture specialist will know which acupuncture point to stimulate based on locating points on the body where stimulation will produce a beneficial change in the central nervous system, which will alter your horse's condition. The number of treatments required depends upon the condition treated and how long the problem has existed. The length of individual treatments usually ranges from 5 to 30 minutes.

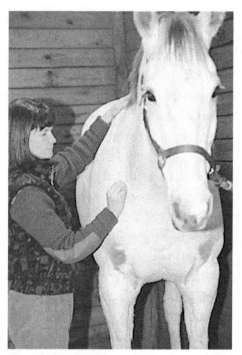

Fig. 26. Dry needle insertion to stimulate accupuncture points.

The Acupuncture Lameness Exam

Acupuncture is an excellent diagnostic aid in addition to your veterinarian's conventional lameness exam. Acupuncture diagnosis is based on the level of sensitivity to palpation of particular acupuncture points (acupoints) that have been found to correspond with specific conditions. There are also diagnostic trigger points (acupoints), knots or tight bands in a muscle, that help the practitioner diagnose the problem. For example, a triceps trigger point is often quite sensitive to palpation when lower leg lameness is present. Diagnostic acupoints may not entirely locate the lameness or its cause, but they do give the practitioner information that reactive points are there. Each diagnostic acupoint may have four or five meanings, depending on which other points are reactive. The combination of reactive points assists your vet's diagnosis. Sometimes acupoint diagnosis will help determine which of two or more problems may have come first, such as in the case of a lower limb lameness accompanied by a back problem.

Acupuncture diagnosis can be an excellent adjunct to the lameness examination in addition to flexion tests, diagnostic nerve blocks, X-rays and ultrasound.

Using Acupuncture to Treat Lameness

Acupuncture is used to treat various injuries, although it is not usually used to treat the primary problem of a tendon or ligament injury. What happens is that once your horse alters his gait from lameness, let's say from a bowed tendon, his back may become sore as a secondary, or compensatory, event and patterns of trigger points in the back or neck may remain unresolved. Acupuncture therapy may then be used quite successfully to treat the secondary problems of the primary tendon or ligament problem. Why treat the secondary problems? Well, once your horse recovers from his tendon or ligament injury, body pain stemming from his injury may prevent him from performing up to his ability. Acupuncture may help that issue. It has been used successfully to treat chronic back problems, hock or stifle problems, laminitis, navicular disease and various soft tissue injuries (see Figure 27). It can also be used to treat colic, diarrhea and reproductive, neurologic and respiratory conditions.

Further research is necessary and will undoubtedly continue to explain the physiologic basis of this ancient technique.

Chiropractic Care

Chiropractic care is a holistic approach to many of the health and performance problems that a horse may have. Although chiropractic care is not typically indicated for treating tendon and ligament injuries, these injuries can cause secondary conditions that may

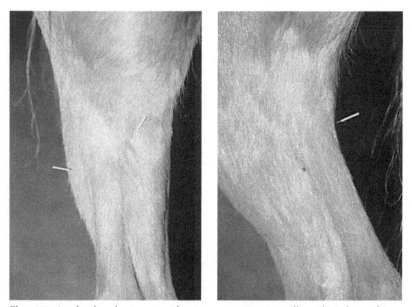

Fig. 27. Look closely to see the accupuncture needles that have been inserted into the horse's rear leg.

warrant chiropractic care. It does not replace traditional veterinary medicine and surgery, but provides an alternative method of care. Chiropractic adjustments are helpful in treating gait abnormalities and other problems that cause poor performance in the athletic horse. It can alleviate pain in your horse's back and neck and alleviate ailments such as pressure on the sciatic nerve. A brief look at what type of care chiropractors give will help show how they can be used if your horse has a tendon or ligament injury.

What Is Chiropractic Care?

Common stressful or traumatic situations in the horse, such as the birth process, poor conformation, training, shoeing abnormalities or direct trauma, can cause abnormal or restricted movement of the spine. The improperly positioned spine that is no longer moving correctly is what chiropractors call a subluxation. When a subluxation occurs, the horse's spine loses its normal flexibility. Subluxations can

---

RESOURCES

To locate a certified veterinary acupuncturist and learn more about equine acupuncture, visit the following Web sites:

International Veterinary Acupuncture Society (IVAS): http://www.ivas.org

American Academy of Veterinary Acupuncture (AAVA): http://www.aava.org

American Academy of Veterinary Medical Acupuncture (AAVMA): http://www.aavma.org

---

cause stiffness, which only makes the problem worse because it leads to resistance and decreased performance. Pain is the most common symptom associated with spinal subluxations. When your horse is in pain, he may change his normal posture and alter his gait, which causes stress in other joints and muscles.

Spinal misalignments, or subluxations, are commonly associated with the following symptoms:

- Lameness

- Stiffness

- Poor attitude

- Muscle atrophy (degeneration)

- Lack of impulsion from behind and difficulty in maintaining collection

- Gait abnormalities

- Being cold-backed or flinchy when his back is touched

Horse owners commonly complain that a horse demonstrates stiffness, resistance to one direction, irritability, decreased performance and touchiness when being groomed.

How May Chiropractic Care Help a Horse with a Tendon or Ligament Injury?

In horses, back problems and leg injuries often go together. When your horse injures his tendon or ligament, he is typically lame. The injury causes him to alter his gait, placing more weight on healthy limbs. The unbalanced weight distribution and altered gait can overwork associated back muscles and increase forces to joints. Ultimately, spinal subluxations occur and the series of problems becomes cyclical. Once the tendon injury is healed, there remains an unresolved issue with your horse's back. This is where chiropractic care may be beneficial (see Figure 28). It should be noted that without proper shoeing and a balanced foot, chiropractic care is of minimal value. As with your own body, many parts have to work together. If one part is off, it affects other parts. It's the same with your horse.

Your veterinary chiropractor can provide the veterinarian additional means of diagnosis and early treatment options in certain lameness problems, especially conservative treatment of biomechanically related musculoskeletal disorders.

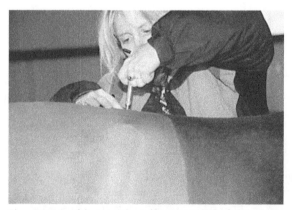

Fig. 28. A chiropractic adjustment of the horse's back muscles, using an activator.

It should be stressed that chiropractic care should in no way replace conventional veterinary medicine. Instead, it should be a complementary treatment procedure for many back and lameness problems. It's important to contact your veterinarian so that he or she can assess your horse for any underlying medical conditions that could be causing similar symptoms.

If your horse has a tendon or ligament injury, he may be predisposed to back or joint problems that may alter his performance even when the initial injury is healed. It's in these cases that a chiropractor may help.

It is important to have your veterinarian refer you to a certified veterinary chiropractor. Certification means that he or she is either a licensed human chiropractor or a veterinarian who has gone through additional training and passed a certification exam. The American Veterinary Chiropractic Association can refer you to a licensed practitioner in your state.

Therapeutic Ultrasound

Diagnostic ultrasound is what veterinarians use to diagnose and monitor tendon and ligament lesions in the horse. Therapeutic ultrasound uses the same sound waves to theoretically treat these same lesions. The sound waves create heat in the tissue and may increase circulation. Although human studies report benefits of therapeutic ultrasound including increased collagen production, decreased scar tissue and enhanced healing, there haven't been many studies in animals. One recent study on the effect of this therapy on the healing of surgically severed Achilles tendons in dogs suggested that the treated animals had less scar tissue and enhanced healing rates. Other older studies have not proven any benefit or have been contradictory. One problem is that researchers have not standardized treatment regimes or dosages. In theory, heat applied to an inflamed tendon using therapeutic ultrasound could make the problem worse. Therefore, if you want to consider this treatment it would be wise to apply it after the inflammatory phase of tendon healing. Review Chapter 3 on the phases of tendon healing.

Low-Level Laser Therapy (Cold or Soft Lasers)

Laser equipment manufacturers claim that laser therapy (a lower level of light than used to cut tissue) increases circulation and thus speeds healing of tendon and ligament injuries and skin wounds. Despite many nonscientific observations, experimental studies have yet to substantiate any benefit. One scientific study found no benefit in horses with tendon injuries. Another found that results in laser-treated horses were less favorable than those horses treated conservatively. Based on this research, laser therapy has not yet shown a benefit in treating tendon or ligament injuries.

Electrical and Electromagnetic Therapy

Electrical and electromagnetic stimulation therapy for tendon and ligament injuries is sometimes used with conventional therapies. Minimal research on the effectiveness of this treatment has been conducted. In some cases, electrical and electromagnetic stimulation may have negative results. One study evaluated the healing of surgically created defects in both front SDF tendons of 20 horses after researchers applied pulsed electromagnetic field therapy (PEMF) to one SDF tendon on each horse for two hours daily. Their results indicate that PEMF significantly delayed tissue maturation at weeks 8 and 12 compared to the limb that did not receive PEMF. One study in rabbit tendons indicated that a continuous electrical current passed through a repair site on a flexor tendon may facilitate collagen formation.

There is simply not enough scientific information to make a conclusion as to PEMF usefulness. The evidence that does exist is negative and, thus, is reason enough to avoid this therapy for tendon or ligament injuries.

Magnetic Therapy

Magnetic boots are quite popular now. Manufacturers claim that these devices improve circulation and thus can improve a variety of conditions afflicting the horse. Again, there is no scientific evidence that magnetic therapy has benefited any horse. However, there are no studies suggesting any harmful effects, either. This seems to be one of those therapies that, even if it isn't beneficial, won't cause harm if you try it.

In Summary

- Not all alternative therapies are harmless.

- Some therapies can delay healing.

- Do your research. If you have any questions about an alternative therapy, discuss it with your veterinarian or do your own research on the Internet, or preferably by calling one of the 27 veterinary schools and speaking with a specialist.

Chapter 9

Preventing Tendon and Ligament Injury

The only thing better than the successful rehabilitation of a tendon or ligament injury is one that never happens. With all that researchers know about these injuries, it is surprising how much we don't know about how to prevent them. However, there are precautions you should take to minimize the chances of your horse incurring one of these serious injuries. Although not guaranteed to prevent an injury, following these guidelines will give you and your horse the best chance for avoiding catastrophe.

Knowing What Normal Looks Like

It cannot be overstated that familiarity with your horse's normal appearance is one of the single best ways to prevent injury. We learned earlier that full-blown tendon injuries typically result from microdamage that occurs over time, damage that is not always readily accessible to the naked eye. Yet, many times, with careful attention, you will be able to pick up on slight "filling" of the leg in the area of the tendon, or maybe a little heat in one leg relative to

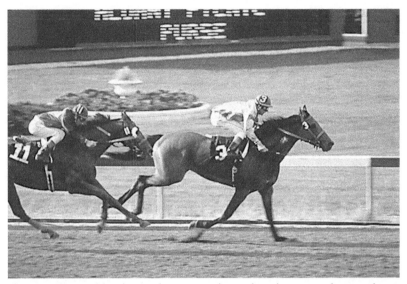

Fig. 29. Thoroughbreds on the racetrack need to be warmed up and not overworked.

the other. Maybe your horse misstepped coming out of his stall or took one or two lame steps, then walked fine. These are all indications that you should consult your veterinarian about. They may indicate that microtrauma has occurred, and it's time to give your horse a break along with a thorough lameness examination. Look and feel your horse's legs every day you see him. Learning to recognize the subtle signs of an injury before it becomes severe is a sure way to prevent worsening.

Proper Footing

Uneven ground, rock-covered surfaces or deep or muddy footing are perfect conditions for predisposing your horse to a tendon or ligament injury. Ideal footing is no more than two to three inches deep and usually composed of angular sand on a base of compacted limestone or decomposed granite. Footing that is too thin offers little concussion protection for your horse. Deep footing adds strain

---

RESOURCES FOR QUALITY EQUINE FOOTING

Under Foot. The USDF Guide to Dressage Arena Construction, Maintenance and Repair. U.S. Dressage Federation, Lexington, Ky., 2000.
"On Sound Footing," *Equus,* October 1993, pp. 30–37.
"Arena Makeover," *Equus,* June 1999, pp. 39–49.

---

to tendons and ligaments. Most footing material protects against concussion best when its moisture content is between 8 percent and 12 percent.

It is best if you can maintain your own arena footing, but this isn't always possible. The footing at your stable or racetrack may be someone else's responsibility. But you, as a user of the facilities, can bring the condition to the attention of the appropriate people. Sometimes this is all that is needed. At least be observant and proactive about where your horse must work. If it's not right, don't ride, even if it means loading your horse in your trailer and heading home from an event or a show.

Conditioning

People sometimes minimize the necessity of proper conditioning before strenuous exercise and many times end up with an injured horse. Not only do the tendons need to become accustomed to a workload, but their connecting muscles must, also. An improperly conditioned muscle becomes fatigued then stiff during a strenuous workout. With less muscle elasticity and support, more stress is placed on tendons, increasing the likelihood of damage. The best approach is to identify your horse's job first. Is he a barrel racer, a reiner, a cutting horse, a roping horse, a racehorse, a jumper or a hunter? Then get the best trainer you can find in that field and have him help you properly condition your horse for his task.

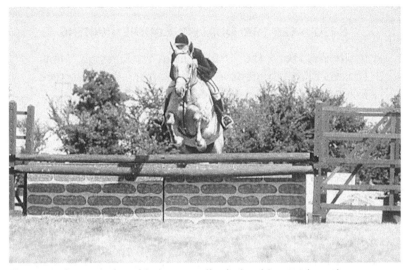

Fig. 30. A hunter takes this jump easily during his round on the course.

The Importance of Warming Up

Just as you can't sprint from your front door for a solid mile at top speed without stiffness and muscle strain, your horse can't, either. Human athletes always warm up prior to a workout. Runners walk a short distance, stretch, then jog slowly for a distance before doing any kind of speed work. Each athletic discipline has its own set of warm-up practices. The athletic horse is the same. He needs an appropriate warm-up before working at his job. This may include walking for at least 10 minutes, then some light jogging, maybe some trotting with long strides or even trotting over ground poles. Depending on your horse's discipline, the warm-up may be different. Some jumping trainers like to walk, then trot, their horses, then start them over small cross-rail jumps, very low to begin with, then work up. Here again, asking a trainer is the best method to ensure that you are doing all you can to properly prepare your horse for his day's work.

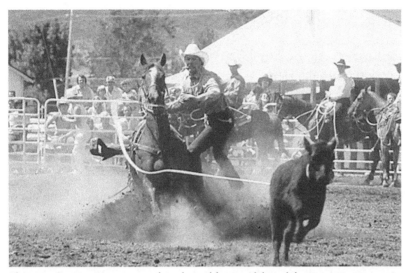

Fig. 31. Quarter Horses need to be athletes with quick moves to compete in roping.

Good Shoeing

One of the most often overlooked areas for preventing injury is your horse's shoeing. Foot imbalance is a major contributor to lameness. Your horse's foot needs to be balanced with a correct foot-pastern angle to minimize unnecessary stress and strain on the soft tissue structures of his legs. Find a good farrier and stick to a rigid timetable of shoeing or trimming every four to eight weeks. It is always best to get referrals for farriers, just as it is for veterinarians. Also, it's always good to know that someone else has had success with a practitioner before your horse sees him. You probably already use the referral method to find doctors for yourself and your family because you feel better when someone you know can recommend the work of someone you don't.

A New Test on the Horizon

Researchers at the Royal Veterinary College at the University of London, Hatfield, Herts, U.K., are working on a new blood test that will diagnose early-stage tendinitis. As discussed in Chapter 3, tendinitis is preceded by tendon degeneration, which is microdamage that occurs over time before the big blow. Racehorses and competition horses may hyperextend and overstress their forelegs a little bit during practice, then a little more during the event, then a little more the following week, but each injury is slight and the horse finds he can ignore it. The owner or trainer may suspect something wrong but can't see any real symptoms. Diagnosing tendon injury at this stage, before your horse is truly lame or has obvious signs, may prevent full-blown bowed tendons.

During tendon degeneration, a protein called cartilage oligomeric matrix protein (COMP) becomes cleaved into fragments and can be found in the horse's blood. Researchers are identifying the cleavage site on the COMP protein specifically involved in tendon degeneration. By developing antibodies to this cleaved product, they are creating a test called an ELISA, or enzyme-linked immunosorbant assay, that will detect the cleaved protein. If your horse tests positive, it would indicate he has tendon damage, even though no one can see it. Your veterinarian and your trainer could then use this information to alter your horse's work schedule and implement a monitoring system and possibly a therapeutic regime that would not only help heal his current subclinical injury but prevent future deterioration into a more serious condition. Although no commercial date has been released, researchers hope the test will soon be available.

Home Safety

Parents of toddlers install gates to prevent their little ones from falling down stairs and remove obstacles from the babies' path to prevent falls. Such should be the life of the conscientious horse owner. Walk your horse's pasture or stall at least once a week to check for sharp metal, deep holes, wire, broken fencing, nails, sharp rocks and other objects that may cause injury. Anything that might lacerate his skin or puncture his foot should be removed. Tendon lacerations are common among horses who stick their legs through broken fences or cracked stall doors, and are preventable by sweeping your eye over his living quarters.

Shipping Safety

Your own experience on the road tells you how rude some drivers can be. While it's easy for you to swerve your car or brake hard and stay securely in your seat, it is another story for a 1,200-pound horse standing in a horse box or a trailer pulled behind a vehicle. It is astounding that there are not more serious accidents in light of the high odds of crashes when you mix horses and cars.

At the very least, braking hard or swerving can cause scrambling feet in an attempt to stay upright in a trailer. It is the equivalent of trying to stand still on a swerving bus. This is why shipping boots or standing wraps that cover your horse's coronary band and stop just below the knee are critical when shipping your horse. Shipping is one area where many coronary lacerations, bruised tendons and general cuts and scrapes are easily preventable, so keep your boots or wraps nearby and don't leave home without them. Horses are like children: it's up to us to make sure we give them the best chance to be injury-free.

In Summary

- Know what your horse's legs look and feel like normally.

- Don't work your horse on improper footing.

- Understand the necessary conditioning work your horse needs for his job.

- Always warm up your horse before working.

- Stick to a rigid shoeing and/or trimming schedule.

- Make sure your horse's living quarters are safe.

- Don't ship your horse without boots or wraps.

Chapter 10

Four Case Studies: Seabiscuit, Mi Bay, Martin and Falcon

Seabiscuit's Journey Back from Suspensory Ligament Desmitis

Seabiscuit was the most famous newsmaker of 1938, getting more newspaper space and radio airtime than Roosevelt, Hitler, Mussolini, Pope Pius XI, Lou Gehrig, Howard Hughes and Clark Gable. He wasn't a pretty racehorse, but he was a fast one, beating out all rivals, including the acclaimed War Admiral. War Admiral had a better pedigree and a wealthier owner, but "the Biscuit," as the public called him, was small, spunky and full of heart. He didn't let War Admiral's long legs, good looks and reputation as a dynamite starter intimidate him. The two horses went nose-to-nose in a specially organized race. Then Seabiscuit simply ran him down, pulling away by several lengths. The crowds loved him.

Beating War Admiral was a great achievement. But for Seabiscuit's California owner, Charles Howard, there was one race that meant more to him than any other: the Santa Anita Handicap,

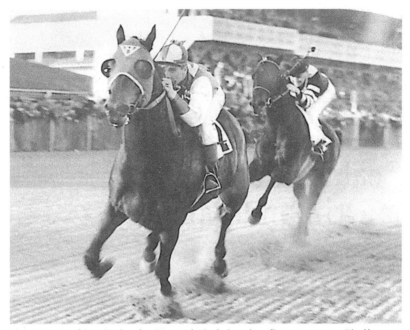

Fig. 32. Seabiscuit leads War Admiral in the first turn at Pimlico on November 1, 1938. Seabiscuit won and set a new track record.

nicknamed the "Hundred-Grander" because that was the purse. It was the one trophy he really wanted Seabiscuit to have.

Laura Hillenbrand wrote in her book about Seabiscuit that the trainer, George Smith, weighed whether running a prep race would be putting too much strain on the horse. But crowds were clamoring to see the Biscuit run, so he was entered in the one-mile Los Angeles Handicap. Halfway through the race, Seabiscuit came down so hard on his left foreleg that the jockey, George Woolf, heard a sharp crack, even above the noise of the race and the crowd.

Woolf tried to pull Seabiscuit up, but the horse fought to keep on going, even though every stride was causing him pain. When he finally slowed down and Woolf jumped off, he saw that the leg appeared structurally normal with no sign of blood. That was the good part. Smith and Howard dashed over to him. Howard led the horse as Smith watched his gait. With every step, Seabiscuit's head nodded. Smith thought it was the horse's ankle.

At the barn, grooms ran for ice, Epson salts and liniment. A groom bandaged Seabicuit's leg in wraps dipped in ice water and sprinkled with Epson salts. Even though the horse was lame, he had to be cooled out after the fast one-mile race he just finished. The track veterinarian examined his leg but couldn't figure out what the injury was. He stated that the injury needed time to declare itself. The vet said that the injury was in the horse's knee and that it could be a broken bone, a blown suspensory ligament or maybe even a little thing like a bruise.

Whatever it was, Howard and Smith didn't waste any time. They took turns all night pouring water on the horse's leg, even while Seabiscut was sleeping. When he awoke, he stood on his bad leg and began eating breakfast. He acted as though nothing was wrong and Howard and Smith hoped against hope that the horse was all right. When they walked him outside in large circles, he didn't limp at all. But when Smith turned the horse sharply to the left, Seabiscuit hobbled.

The veterinarian took X-rays that showed no broken bones. That meant Smith was right: it was the suspensory ligament; one of the worst kinds of injuries for a racehorse. But, whether it was ruptured or just bruised remained to be seen.

Seabiscuit was treated with great care, and soon showed no sign of lameness. His team concluded he must have bruised a suspensory ligament. But when the horse got back on the track for a workout, the worst happened. Seabiscuit once again bobbed his head and limped. Now they knew his suspensory ligament had ruptured. He wouldn't make it to the "Hundred-Grander."

Seabiscuit recuperated at the Howard's ranch, first resting, then taking long walks in the meadow. The walks turned into mounted walks led by another horse and rider. Within a few months the walk turned to a smooth lope. With no sign of lameness, the jockey and owner continued to condition Seabiscuit for another try at the

Santa Anita Handicap. After months of additional conditioning and waiting out the California rains, Seabiscuit came in third in his first race since his injury, but he was sound, which was all Howard and Smith cared about. After several more races, he finally entered and ran the Santa Anita Handicap. Nearing the finish, nose for nose with another horse, Kayak, the jockey held him there stride for stride, and then asked Seabiscuit for more.

Seabiscuit bounded over the track, his spunky little heart pumping his stumpy little legs. Seventy-eight thousand fans went crazy. Seabiscuit claimed the prize that had eluded him up till then.

Seabiscuit's story is quite incredible, as a snapped suspensory ligament is most often a career-ending injury for a racehorse. The patience and care of his owners, his trainer and his jockey are what brought him back from a drastic injury. His recovery took almost an entire year. That was in 1939. Even now, many years later, with dozens more diagnostic and treatment tools at our disposal, it still takes that long to recover. Medicine has changed, but suspensory ligaments have not.

Mi Bay in His New Career

His name was Mi Bay, and he was a paddler. When he moved, as soon as his left front leg came off the ground to move forward, it would paddle out in an arc, like the oar of a boat, before landing. It was most noticeable if you stood directly in front or behind him and watched his legs at any gait. It was striking to watch because it was a lot of extra movement. But extra movement is not efficient. It wastes energy.

Mi Bay was a beauty with a glimmering seal brown coat. He had a way of catching your eye. You couldn't miss him in a crowd. But if you did, you might notice him when the horses moved off toward the starting gate, because of the funny way he walked. Sometimes, farriers wanted to try to straighten out his gait by making him shoes that were higher on the outside or heavier on the inside, or whatever their theory was. But he was born that way and there was no changing him. He was lucky to have owners who understood that.

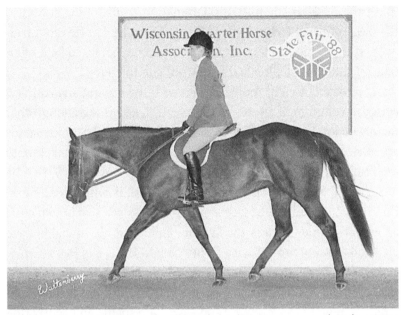

Fig. 33. Bowed tendon ends Mi Bay's racing career . . . but he starts another.

Bay was a racing Quarter Horse, winner of the Shu Fly Handicap at Los Alamitos with lifetime race earnings of $96,848. That's not a lot of money relative to a racing Thoroughbred, but for a Quarter Horse it was something to brag about. He was at least paying the feed and training bills of his owners, at least until the night he broke down right before the finish line and limped off the dirt track on three legs.

Bay's owner and trainer took one look and knew immediately that the horse had bowed his left front leg at the mid–cannon bone region, the leg he paddled. The time was the 1980s, and veterinarians didn't have diagnostic ultrasound to show them exactly what was going on inside a horse's leg. Vets and trainers cared for bowed tendons by old medicine means: cold water hosing, poultice, standing wraps, anti-inflammatory drugs and many times by pin firing. So it was this regime, without the pin firing, that Bay's owner and trainer started. The value of controlled exercise was not known at that time, so after the initial inflammation and swelling subsided, Bay was returned to his owner's farm, where he ran free in a paddock. It was a big paddock and he was a happy horse, so he'd often take off into a full gallop and race from end to end.

It took about eight months, even with the playing and running episodes common of an ex–race horse, to heal his leg enough that he was no longer lame. In most race stables it would be unusual for an owner to keep a nonracing gelding around. After all, horses aren't cheap and Bay certainly wasn't making any money. But he was special. Not only was he strikingly beautiful, with a long neck, thin throatlatch, chiseled face and a summer-sleek seal brown coat, he was also kind. He was the favorite and he would probably have died had a young pre-vet student not caught the eye of Bay's owner.

The student, who was on spring break, offered to ride Bay just to get him out for a little exercise. Every day for five days, she would saddle him up in western gear and a working snaffle and gently ride him in a large arena. There was no sign of lameness and Bay seemed happy to have a job again. After some initial confusion, the horse gave in to the slower approach. Before, once a rider was on his back, he was expected to take off as fast as he could. But he learned to drop his head, jog smoothly and lope slowly around the ring. A bond grew between Bay and the student. It was soon evident to everyone. At the end of the week, the owners invited the student to their home. They told her how much they loved Bay and wanted only the best for him. But now, they felt the best thing would be for him to be with her. They offered to give her their favorite horse. No money, no strings attached, just the expectation that she would take care of him, love him and give him a good home for the rest of his life. And so began Mi Bay's new career.

Bay's new owner trained him first for Hunter Under Saddle, then Western Pleasure, and showed him on the local Quarter Horse Circuit. After many top five finishes, he went on to win High Point Awards in both of his events for two years. For something different, they went team penning at a local barn every Wednesday night and trail riding on Fridays. Bay excelled in both.

This is an example of how a bowed tendon can change a horse's life. Bay was no longer flashing through a finish line. He did not hear the roar of the crowd. His pace was slower. He got a lot more days off. But once healed, the bowed tendon didn't stop him from living a very full life. He still had a career he enjoyed. In fact, his bowed tendon was the thing that led him to me. I don't think either one of us would have wanted to miss out on all the joy we shared during those years.

Martin, the Quarter Horse, Winning the Grand Championship

The Santa Barbara sun shone bright on the early morning workout of hundreds of horses at one of the largest week-long open shows on the California circuit. Martin, an eight-year-old brown Quarter Horse, and Megan, his sixteen-year-old rider, walked briskly around the watered arena amidst many other horses. There were so many horses that you had to pay careful attention to getting on and off the rail or doing any circle work in the middle for fear of getting clobbered. Megan's class wasn't until after lunch, enough time for a morning workout and then stall rest before warming up.

The young girl took Martin through his typical warm-up: ten minutes of fast walking and slow jogging for two laps and then a little more walking. She began a gentle lope, hugging the rail but going around slower moving horses. All seemed fine until she started to move off the rail and looked back to see a runaway horse at their right flank. It was too late. The huge Palomino slammed his shoulder into Martin's hindquarters, causing him to jump sideways, slamming not only the rail horse but then eventually into the rail. Two men at the other end of the arena caught the Palomino.

Everyone was trying to get back to normal. Martin had scrambled, but seemed fine now and Megan continued his workout. Besides dodging the faster horses, all seemed okay. It wasn't until the second slow lope lap that Megan realized something was wrong.

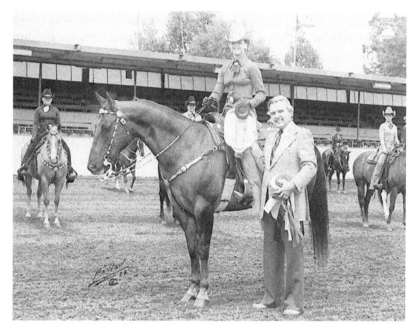

Fig. 34. Martin, the case of the bruised suspensory ligament.

Martin seemed "off." Megan knew her mount and tried to sense how he was feeling through her hands and legs and seat, but couldn't quite pinpoint it. Megan took him over to the rail where her trainer was standing and asked her to watch him trot. Martin's injury became obvious to both of them: he was mildly lame on his left front leg. It was mostly evident at the trot. He walked normally and only seemed a tiny bit off at a canter. But trotting, he was definitely lame.

The trainer asked Megan to dismount. They walked Martin back to the barn and examined his leg. There was nothing to see. Not even any heat. But Martin's trainer did notice that when she palpated his suspensory ligament at one point Martin flinched on that leg but not the other. She decided to call the show veterinarian. After a thorough lameness exam, with flexion tests and full palpation, the vet confirmed that Martin had lightly bruised his suspensory ligament, probably during the scrambling in the arena. The veterinarian suggested anti-inflammatory drugs, cold water hosing and wraps. They decided to scratch the horse from the day's events and monitor his progress.

Of course, on the anti-inflammatory drugs, Martin was not lame at all, but that didn't mean his injury had healed. On day two of his injury, Martin's trainer took him off the anti-inflammatories to determine if he was still lame. Would they have to scratch him from the entire show? It was illegal to show him while the drugs were being administered. On day three, they trotted him in the barn aisle and patiently watched every step. To their relief, they saw no lameness.

They could show him in the remaining events, but they would alter their normal routine. Rather than doing twice-a-day workouts, they carefully monitored short workouts prior to each class. If they saw no lameness, Martin would be allowed to enter his class for the day. It was the year-end championship with two western equitation classes left and then the final grand championship equitation. They all held their breath before the first class. Martin was fine so Megan entered, along with some twenty or so others.

Megan and the trainer thought the class would be fairly fast, therefore limiting the time Martin would have to work. But they were wrong. Twenty minutes went by, and still the judge was picking and choosing. But Martin showed no sign of lameness.

Young Megan prayed silently that Martin would hold up without being hurt. The trainer dug her fingernails into the rail and prayed for the class to be over. Finally, the announcer told the class to walk and bring their horses to the center and line up. Two minutes later, out of one of the largest classes they had ever competed in, the announcer called number 224. The line of riders stood there looking around for 224 to step out. Megan's hand flew to her mouth. She couldn't believe it; after all they had gone through, all the worry and wonder if they were even going to be able to ride, her lost training time and the stress of his injury—they had won!

Megan walked over to the ribbon holder, who held up a large silver tray with a blue ribbon for the photographer. The cameraman shook a can of rocks, Martin's ears flew forward and the flash went off. Megan and Martin went on in that show to win their next class, and then the grand championship.

At the end of the day, Megan gave Martin a hug and told him he was the most wonderful horse in the world, and he gave her a look that said, Why had she ever doubted it? Martin was never lame again.

This is an example of a truly happy story. Sometimes, a small injury develops into a big one. In this case, the fact that the rider and trainer were alert and treated the horse immediately probably went a long way toward ensuring the horse's recovery.

Falcon, the Endurance Champion

Falcon is a mustang. He was born wild in the mountains of the American West. He was captured at three years old and trained to be a competitive endurance horse. Before Falcon injured his right hind leg, he had finished 850 competitive miles (50 miles per competition) over four years, with finishes in the top ten a number of times. If you counted up all the miles that went into his training and conditioning, the figure would be in the thousands. All those miles and he had never once come up lame.

The next event was different. Looking back, Donna, his owner and trainer, concluded that he injured himself during a strong gallop up a long, steep hill on leaf-covered, wet ground, where he slipped and hyper-extended his right rear fetlock joint. At the third vet check, at the 38-mile marker, he was approved to continue the event. But as he trotted out, Donna felt one of his steps go "off." She pulled him up because she knew he wasn't right. She didn't want to take the chance of injuring a beloved horse who had already done so much winning.

Falcon was not really lame. So Donna delayed a diagnostic ultrasound for two weeks because all he showed was a slightly guarded stride for a few steps when turned out during a break after

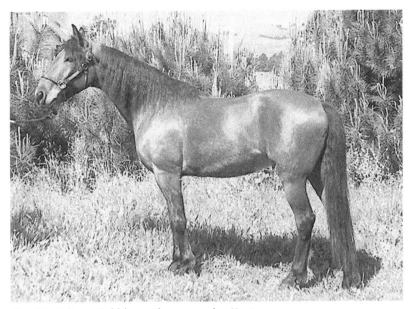

Fig. 35. Falcon: Cold laser therapy and a Mustang.

the competition. She gave Falcon oral anti-inflammatories and rubbed DMSO on his ankle. However, when some slight heat and swelling in the ankle did not subside, she called her veterinarian. A diagnostic ultrasound showed a tear in the deep digital flexor tendon and a small lateral sesamoid bone fracture.

After six weeks of stall rest, the veterinarian suggested that Falcon be shod in full egg bar—a shoe shaped like an egg to offer more heel support—and start a controlled exercise program of riding at a walk for 30 minutes per day, increasing by 5 minutes per week. Donna also started immediately using the Bio-Scan light therapy hock/ankle boots for approximately 20 minutes, twice daily. The light therapy system delivers therapeutic photon and pulsed magnetic field energy to the injured site. She continued the light/laser therapy for three months with definite improvement in Falcon's condition.

Donna thought the light therapy was helping; Falcon improved faster in his right hind leg until he went "off" in the other hind leg. X-rays showed a fractured sesamoid. Falcon not only had three small chip fractures, but an osteochondritis desicans (OCD) lesion in his ankle as well. OCD lesions are developmental and predispose the area to degeneration, leading to lameness. Donna was sure that it was Falcon's compensation for these unknown lesions in his left hind that helped create his initial injury in his right hind leg.

With nine months of reduced work and light therapy on both ankles Falcon finally healed enough to start working again. But, with his OCD lesion it was too risky to return him to endurance racing. He has remained sound as a school and dressage horse, working on flat ground for the past three years.

Scientific research on the efficacy on light/laser therapy on healing rates in horses is slow but ongoing. There is quite a bit of anecdotal evidence that this therapy helps horses heal faster with little or no evidence of any adverse side effects. In this case, it is probably one of those therapies that is okay to try. If it helps, great. Donna Snyder-Smith feels it helped Falcon significantly, and she recommends it to other riders.

Bibliography

Chan, W., C. Kuang-Yang, H. Liu, L. Wu, and J. Lin. "Acupuncture for general veterinary practice." *Journal of Veterinary Medical Science* 63 *(*2001): 1057–1062.

Dowling, B. A., A. J. Dart, D. R. Hodgson, and R. K. Smith. "Superficial digital flexor tendonitis in the horse." *Equine Veterinary Journal* 32 *(*2000): 368–378.

Hillenbrand, Laura. *Seabiscuit: An American Legend.* New York: Random House. 2001.

Reef, V. B. "Superficial digital flexor tendon healing: Ultrasonographic evaluation of therapies." *The Veterinary Clinics of North America Equine Practice* 17 (2001): 159–178.

Saini, N. S., K. S. Roy, P. S. Bansal, B. Singh, and P. S. Simran. "A preliminary study on the effect of ultrasound therapy on healing of surgically severed Achilles tendons in five dogs." *Journal of Veterinary Medicine Series A, Physiology, Pathology, Clinical Medicine.* 49 (2002): 321–328.

Stashak, T. *Adams' Lameness in Horses.* 5th ed. Philadelphia: Lippincott Williams & Wilkins, 2002.

Watkins, J. P., J. A. Auer, S. J. Morgan, and S. Gay. "Healing of surgically created defects in the equine superficial digital flexor tendon:
Effects of pulsing electromagnetic field therapy on collagen-type
transformation and tissue morphologic reorganization."
American Journal of Veterinary Research 46 (1985): 2097–2103.

Resources

Useful Internet Web Sites

The following is a list of Internet Web sites you might find useful. For more information, do your own inquiry on an Internet search engine, as articles, information, and Web sites appear and disappear frequently.

American Association of Equine Practitioners: www.aaep.org

American College of Veterinary Internal Medicine: www.acvim.org

American Veterinary Medical Association: www.avma.org

Equine Health Articles by Randy Sublett: www.wiwfarm.com/sublett.htm

Horses @ Purdue: www.vet.purdue.edu/horses

Leg Injuries in Horses: www.leg-injuries-in-horses.com

Spirits on the Hoof: www.pets-therapy.com/Equine/Spirits-On-The-Hoof.htm

The Horse: www.thehorse.com

UC Davis: Diagnostic Ultrasound & Musculoskeletal Injuries in Horses: www.vmth.ucdavis.edu/vmth/clientinfo/info/laus/lausbroch.html

Vetgate: vetgate.ac.uk

Books

The following books offer useful additional information regarding care of the injured horse, and training and conditioning to prevent injuries.

The All-Around Horse and Rider, Donna Snyder-Smith

A number of major innovations in horse handling have gained acceptance in the past years. This book helps amateur adult riders understand the new approaches and new riding techniques and implement them. With her strong competition background, the author has good advice to increase the strength and endurance of both horse and rider, much of which appeared in her first book, *The Complete Guide to Endurance Riding and Competition.*

A–Z of Horse Diseases & Health Problems, Tim Hawcroft

This book provides detailed descriptions of equine diseases and includes photographs and a detailed index. It gives the owner instant access to disease symptoms and signs, diagnoses, causes, and treatments, as well as basic first aid. (He doesn't deal with tendon and ligament injuries, as those are not diseases.)

Consumer's Guide to Alternative Therapies in the Horse, David W. Ramey

The author sorts through misconceptions and myths surrounding alternative therapies chapter by chapter, and what science has discovered about them. He evaluates acupuncture, manual therapy, massage, homeopathy, energy medicine, herbal therapy, laser and light therapy, magnetic therapy and others.

Equine Massage: A Practical Guide, Jean-Pierre Hourdebaigt

The author, a Registered Massage Therapist who works on performance horses in all sports, explains to owners and trainers how they can use massage to deal with injuries during training or competition. He covers anatomy and physiology, principles and concepts of massage, and gives a stretching and check-up routine. The book is illustrated with diagrams and step-by-step sequences of photographs.

The Essentials of Horsemanship: Training, Riding, Care and Management, Jocelyn Drummond

Horses are complex and sensitive creatures who can be upset by inappropriate feeding, poorly fit saddles, too much or too little exercise, all of which can make them uncomfortable and possibly sick. The author gives basic information about horses and and how to keep them. All the information here fosters a better understanding of the horse, his nature and his needs.

Horse Gaits, Balance and Movement, Susan E. Harris

This book is full of important information on the biomechanics of balance in the horse. It teaches the rider to maximize the horse's athletic ability and minimize the chance of injury. The author has written several other important manuals for the United States Pony Club.

Horse Owner's Veterinary Handbook, 2nd Edition, James M. Giffin, Tom Gore

This reference work by two veterinarians is the kind of helpful book you want on your shelf. It communicates the information owners need to maintain their horse's health. It addresses basic health-care and management issues such as the latest medicines and immunizations, wounds, illnesses, parasites, nutrition and supplements, and reproduction.

Training Strategies for Dressage Riders, Charles de Kunffy

De Kunffy examines dressage as an art form, while giving riders training strategies to improve the partnership with their horses. These strategies include exercises for suppling, strengthening and correcting the horse. It offers a complete training system for both horse and rider, paying special attention to how a rider's actions can influence a mount. In this book, de Kunffy continues his previous work, *The Athletic Development of the Dressage Horse.*

The USPC Guide to Bandaging Your Horse, Susan E. Harris, Ruth Ring Harvie, eds.

The USPC Guide provides information about bandaging, leg care, and keeping your horse's legs sound. It explains the many kinds of bandages and bandage materials available, their purposes, and when to use them. There are detailed drawings and step-by-step instructions on how to apply bandages for shipping, stable, exercise, and various treatments. It provides tips on the best types of materials to use.

The USPC Guide to Conformation, Movement and Soundness, Susan E. Harris

The United States Pony Club Guide to Conformation, Movement and Soundness explains and illustrates functional conformation and movement, conformation defects, faulty movement, unsoundnesses, the causes, and how they affect the horse. This guide will be helpful to anyone interested in learning about evaluating conformation, soundness and way of moving.

Ultimate Horse Care: The Complete Veterinary Guide, John McEwen, ed.

Ultimate Horse Care focuses on practical horse care, from common ailments to alternative methods of treatment. It focuses attention on how horses function and how to improve their quality of life.

Magazines

Here are some resources in which you will find articles keeping up with the latest in treatments and therapies for injured horses, and information on conditioning, training, and nutrition.

Arabian Horse World
    This magazine promotes the Arabian horse with articles about breeding and showing and racing this beautiful breed. Features on photography and breeding programs.
    www.ahwmagazine.com
    (800) 955-9423

Dressage Today
    Devoted exclusively to the sport and art of dressage, one of America's most popular equestrian disciplines. It features insights

from the world's most respected trainers, riders, and judges. It includes coverage of national and international dressage events, as well as articles on the care and management of dressage horses.

www.equisearch.com.

Equus

This magazine provides the latest information from top veterinarians, equine researchers, riders and trainers on understanding and influencing equine behavior, recognizing the warning signs of illness and disease, and solving riding and training problems.

www.equusmagazine.com

(800) 829-5910

Horse Illlustrated: The Magazine for Responsible Horse Owners

Horse Illustrated is a magazine of interest to all sports and disciplines, with articles on health care, nutrition, behavior, riding, grooming, training, and profiles of different breeds.

www.horseillustratedmagazine.com

(800) 365-4421

Horse & Rider: The Authority on Western Riding and Training

In every issue there are articles on training by experts, the latest on equine health care, trail riding tips, the essentials of hands-on horse care.

www.horseandrider.com

(877) 717-8928

Practical Horseman

A magazine for English riders of all disciplines. It adopts a "how-to" approach in its articles, such as step by-step training programs, money- and time-saving ideas on health care and stable management, and advice from recognized experts in hunters, jumpers, equitation, dressage, and eventing.

www.equisearch.com.

Q: The American Quarter Horse Journal

The American Quarter Horse Association calls their breed "America's Horse" and supports them with registries, shows, and magazines devoted to the care, health, competition, breeding and maintenance of quality of Quarter horses.

www.aqha.com

(800) 291-7323

Thoroughbred Times

A weekly newsmagazine based in Lexington, Kentucky, written for those involved in Thoroughbred racing and breeding and for racing fans. They publish an annual *Stallion Directory* and *Auction Review*, which reports on all horses sold or offered at public auction in North America.

www.thoroughbredtimes.com

1-888-499-9090

Picture Credits

Photos pp. 7, 14, 15, 43, 49, 50, 54, courtesy of Mary Beth Whitcomb, DVM, University of California-Davis, School of Veterinary Medicine, Davis, Calif.; pp. 12, 36, 61, courtesy of Steve Trostle DVM, MS, Diplomate ACVS, San Luis Rey Equine Hospital, Bonsall, Calif.; p. 20, reprinted with permission from Photobysparks.com, Deanna Sparks-Kjorlien Photography; p. 35, Peri Hughes, courtesy of Equine Research, Inc.; p. 55 by Caitlin Wallace of Competitor 3, Andalusian owned by Stephane Simon; pp. 80, 81, 84, by Allison M. Howell, DVM; p. 98, Associated Press; p. 106, by Donna Snyder-Smith

Index